Locoregional Treatment Considerations in Early Breast Cancer

Frederick L. Moffat, Jr., M.D., F.A.C.S., F.R.C.S.(C)

University of Miami School of Medicine
Miami, Florida U.S.A.

R.G. Landes Company
Austin

MEDICAL INTELLIGENCE UNIT

LOCOREGIONAL TREATMENT CONSIDERATIONS IN EARLY BREAST CANCER

R.G. LANDES COMPANY
Austin

CRC Press is the exclusive worldwide distributor of publications of the Medical Intelligence Unit.
CRC Press, 2000 Corporate Blvd., NW, Boca Raton, FL 33431. Phone: 407/994-0555.

Submitted: April 1994
Published: June 1994

Production Manager: Deborah Molsberry
Acquisitions Editor: Karen Ross
Copy Editor: Susanne Grosch

Please address all inquiries to the Publisher:
R.G. Landes Company, 909 Pine Street, Georgetown, TX 78626
or
P.O. Box 4858, Austin, TX 78765
Phone: 512/ 863 7762; FAX: 512/ 863 0081

ISBN 1-57059-087-7
CATALOG # LN9087

While the authors, editors and publisher believe that drug selection and dosage and the specifications and usage of equipment and devices, as set forth in this book, are in accord with current recommendations and practice at the time of publication, they make no warranty, expressed or implied, with respect to material described in this book. In view of the ongoing research, equipment development, changes in governmental regulations and the rapid accumulation of information relating to the biomedical sciences, the reader is urged to carefully review and evaluate the information provided herein.

Library of Congress Cataloging–in–Publication Data

Moffat, Frederick L.
    Locoregional treatment considerations in early breast cancer /
Frederick L. Moffat, Jr.
        p. cm. — (Medical intelligence unit)
    Includes bibliographical references and index.
    ISBN 1-57059-087-7 (hardcover)
    1. Breast — Cancer — Treatment. 2. Breast — Cancer — Surgery.
I. Title. II. Series.
    [DNLM: 1. Breast Neoplasms — therapy. WP 870 M695L 1994]
RC280.B8M58 1994
616.99'44906 — dc20
DNLM/DLC
for Library of Congress   94-12632
                                                                      CIP

To Our Readers

R.G. Landes Company publishes four book series: *Medical Intelligence Unit, Molecular Biology Intelligence Unit, Neuroscience Intelligence Unit,* and *Biotechnology Intelligence Unit.* Our goal is to publish the most recent information in biomedical science for sophisticated researchers and physicians.

To achieve this goal we have accelerated our publishing program to conform to the fast pace in which information grows in biomedical science. The book you have in hand, like all titles in our series, was published *within 90 days of receipt of the manuscript.*

As you might expect, this causes a few problems for us; sometimes it makes our office more like a big city newspaper than a scholarly publisher. So as you look through this book you may see something that isn't just right. Please let us know. Or if you have an idea for improving our books, we'd like very much to hear from you. If the problem you describe hasn't already been discovered or if your idea is provocative enough to promote a discussion here, we'll give you a free book of your choice. Just list three titles in order of preference and we'll send you one, based on availability—with our thanks. Our address is printed on the copyright page of each of our books.

Elinda McKenna
Director of Operations
R.G. Landes Company

To Alfred S. Ketcham, M.D., who as mentor, surgical oncologist and friend is such an inspiration and source of strength to his colleagues, fellows, residents and students.

CONTENTS

Despite the sustained and innovative efforts of basic and clinical researchers over the past 40 years, breast cancer remains one of the foremost causes of morbidity and death among women in western societies. Recognition that adenocarcinoma of the breast becomes a systemic disease at a preclinical stage in its natural history has been long in coming. The acceptance of breast-conserving therapy as equivalent to radical surgery for Stage I and II disease represents a signal advance in the oncology community's approach to cancer management.

This fundamental change in treatment philosophy was prompted by the realization that ever more radical cancer operations do not eventuate in improved cure rates for many solid tumors. Moreover, the functional, aesthetic, psychological and psychosexual morbidity of many such surgical procedures are formidable. In the absence of clear evidence of locoregional treatment-related improvements in survival, the focus of attention in oncology has widened to include both cancer control and quality of life.

Breast conservation is perhaps the prototypical example of this change in approach to the treatment of malignant disease. The efficacy of breast-conserving therapy has been established at a time when the doctor-patient relationship is changing rapidly, particularly with respect to informed consent and patient autonomy. Patients with early breast cancer now have at least two standard treatment options to choose from. Physicians are therefore obliged to educate patients and take their philosophical perspectives into account to a degree that would have seemed inappropriate and irrelevant to breast cancer management not so long ago.

This monograph is focused on recent developments in the locoregional management of breast cancer. Many questions remain unresolved in this area. This is reflected in the myriad therapeutic regimens in use worldwide which qualify as breast-conserving therapy, uncertainties regarding the significance and treatment of in situ carcinoma, and differences of opinion regarding the management of the axilla and opposite breast, to name only a few ongoing controversies.

In addressing breast conservation in early breast cancer, it has been my foremost objective to present a reasonably comprehensive and balanced treatment of the subject. Inevitably, readers may take issue with some of the points made in this work; this is as it should be, as there is ample room for legitimate differences of opinion in matters pertaining to locoregional breast cancer treatment. The views expressed here are mine, although they also reflect in part the perspectives and practices of the Division of Surgical Oncology at the University of Miami.

In writing a monograph on as broad a subject as locoregional breast cancer treatment, the scope of discussion must be circumscribed to some degree. Accordingly, I have chosen not to address recent developments in breast reconstruction because of this book's focus on breast conservation, and because reconstructive surgery is a broad field in and of itself. In addition, the recent political and medicolegal controversies surrounding breast implants preclude succinct consideration of this topic. With regret, I have discussed only briefly the issue of preoperative adjuvant chemotherapy for locally advanced breast cancer because this volume deals primarily with early breast cancer. Recent results with preoperative chemotherapy for Stage III breast carcinoma may have exciting implications for locoregional management of Stage I and II disease in the future.

With these caveats and restrictions, recent developments in locoregional breast cancer treatment are presented here.

Addendum

The issue of scientific fraud involving patient accrual to the National Surgical Adjuvant Breast and Bowel Project (NSABP) breast cancer protocols from one participating institution first came to light only days after the completed manuscript for this book had been submitted to the publisher. The National Cancer Institute (NCI) and the NSABP have since undertaken extensive audits of the B-06, B-13 and B-14 trials, these being the studies directly affected by proven scientific misconduct. More extensive reviews are in progress or are planned.

Dr. Bernard Fisher and the NSABP have reanalyzed these three trials after exclusion of all patients from the offending institution, and have confirmed the original conclusions. Most appropriately, it has been emphasized by the NCI, other governmental agencies and many distinguished clinical researchers that the conclusions of these and other NSABP studies are corroborated by the results of prospective clinical trials worldwide.[1,2] Thus, my extensive references to NSABP data and conclusions do not necessitate revising this book or delaying its publication. The NSABP studies remain among the most rigorous and scientifically informative clinical breast cancer trials ever conducted.

The magnificent achievements of the NSABP and its founding Chairman may have been temporarily overshadowed by this most unfortunate turn of events. However, in the long run as in the past, the work of Dr. Fisher and his group will continue to be cited and honored for its integrity and enormous significance.

References

1. NCI issues information on falsified data in NSABP trials. J Natl. Cancer Inst 1994; 84:487-489.
2. Angell M, Kassirer JP. Setting the record straight in the breast-cancer trials. New Engl J Med 1994; 330:1448-1450.

Acknowledgements

I am most indebted to Dr. Carolyn Mies, Assistant Professor of Pathology and Dr. Joyce Lentz, Associate Professor of Clinical Radiology for taking time from their busy schedules to assist me in the preparation of this monograph. Dr. Mies selected and photographed the histopathology figures, and Dr. Lentz selected the radiographs for this work. Their contributions have added much to this discussion of early breast cancer and are enormously appreciated.

CHAPTER 1

Conservative Treatment of Breast Cancer
Historical Perspective and Current Status

Breast cancer has been the focus of much attention in medical writings since earliest recorded history. The Egyptians, the classical Greeks and mediaeval Arabs all left documentation of the prevalence and treatment of breast diseases in their place and time, the available therapy usually consisting of surgical excision, cautery or a combination of the two.[1] Although ignorance of the nature and behavior of malignant breast disease remained profound until modern times, a number of early medical practitioners made mention of the importance of excision through normal tissues beyond the periphery of the breast cancer.[1-3]

With the advent of anaesthesia, surgical asepsis and histopathological diagnosis, meticulous control of bleeding, prevention of perioperative infection and radical resection of malignant disease became possible for the first time.[3] Surgery had previously been a crude undertaking carried out with utmost haste because of the unspeakable pain borne by the unanaesthetized patient.[4] The discovery of the efficacy of ionizing radiations in treatment of malignant neoplasia was also a major breakthrough, although truly effective, relatively nontoxic radiotherapy awaited the development of the field of radiation biology and megavoltage technology.

RADICAL BREAST CANCER SURGERY

William Halsted's radical mastectomy was the embodiment of the first rational approach to treatment of breast cancer. Halsted regarded adenocarcinoma of the breast as an exclusively locoregional problem early in its course, spreading to distant sites through an orderly, predictable progression from the primary tumor through the first and second echelon regional lymph nodes. This philosophy provided the rationale for en bloc resection of involved supraclavicular lymph nodes, although the grave prognosis of supraclavicular lymphatic metastases was clearly evident in his own experience as presented to the American Surgical Association in 1907.[5]

In reporting his results with radical mastectomy in 210 breast cancer patients, Halsted noted that 75% of 60 patients with disease confined to the breast remained disease-free at five years' followup, as compared to 31% of the 110 patients with axillary metastases and 10% of 40 patients with axillary and supraclavicular node involvement.[5]

Spread of breast cancer to distant sites from regional lymph nodes was thought to occur via the lymphatics of the superficial and deep fascia of the body. Brain metastases were attributed to spread via the lymphatics accompanying the middle meningeal artery. This concept led to his advocacy of en bloc excision of the fascia of the rectus abdominis, serratus anterior, latissimus dorsi, subscapularis and teres major muscles, and wide excision of the skin of the breast. Halsted's intellectual approach to the surgical management of breast cancer eventually found its most aggressive expression in the extended or super-radical mastectomies, which included en bloc resection of the internal mammary and supraclavicular lymphatics and even sections of the bony thorax.[6-8]

THE RETREAT FROM RADICAL SURGERY FOR EARLY BREAST CANCER

In 1948 Patey and Dyson[9] proposed that removal of the pectoral muscles might not be important for local or systemic control of breast cancer. Noting the relatively sparse lymphatic drainage of the pectoralis fascia as compared to the rich dermal lymphatic plexus in the breast skin, they reported a comparison of the Halsted operation to their "modified radical mastectomy" from their experience at the Middlesex Hospital, London. Their operation included generous en bloc resection of the nipple and breast skin with the breast parenchyma and pectoralis major fascia, but left the pectoral muscles and their innervation intact. There were no differences in survival or cure related to these operations. These results were corroborated in a subsequent report[10] which also included a few cases managed by simple mastectomy plus axillary radiotherapy, and partial mastectomy. Patey concluded that the course of the disease was little affected by en bloc resection of the breast and underlying musculature, while the functional and cosmetic advantages of pectoral muscle preservation were considerable. By the 1970s the Patey operation had supplanted Halsted's mastectomy in the United Kingdom, the British Commonwealth countries and parts of the United States.

Robert McWhirter published the experience with total mastectomy plus radiation to the axillary and supraclavicular nodes (3750 rad in three weeks) from the Royal Infirmary in Edinburgh. Like those of Patey, his observations called into question the rationale for radical mastectomy.[11,12] In making the case for less radical treatment, McWhirter reasoned that mastectomy had been clearly shown to control breast cancer limited to the primary site, and this justified its continued use. In contrast, axillary lymphadenectomy had been of little therapeutic value in breast cancer patients as measured by survival data available at the time. Removal of uninvolved axillary lymphatics obviously could not be of any therapeutic benefit, and primary resection of cancer-bearing axillary nodes failed to prevent death from distant disease in most cases. He speculated that surgical disturbance of involved axillary nodes might even facilitate breast cancer dissemination. His results with "simple" mastectomy and regional nodal irradiation between 1941 and 1945 were superior to those achieved with radical mastectomy at his institution prior to that time.[11]

In 1971, the National Surgical Adjuvant Breast and Bowel Project (NSABP) began accrual to the B-04 prospective randomized trial of patients with clinical node-negative (cN-) and clinical node-positive (cN+) breast cancer. The purpose of this trial was to determine whether in cN- patients total mastectomy alone (with delayed axillary lymphadenectomy only in the event of interval development of palpable nodal metastases) was as effective as radical mastectomy, whether total mastectomy plus regional nodal irradiation was as effective as radical mastectomy, and whether total mastectomy alone was comparable in terms of survival to total mastectomy plus nodal irradiation. Among cN+ patients, radical mastectomy and total mastectomy plus nodal irradiation were compared.

At ten years followup, there were no differences in survival, disease-free survival or distant disease-free survival among the

Table 1.1. Ten-year results of the NSABP B-04 trial[13]

| | cN− Breast Cancer Patients | | | cN+ Breast Cancer Patients | |
	Rad. Mast.	Tot. Mast.	Tot. Mast. plus rXRT	Rad. Mast.	Tot. Mast. plus rXRT
No. Patients	362	352	365	292	294
Disease-free Survival	47 ± 3%	42 ±3%	48 ± 3% p = 0.2	29 ± 3%	25 ± 3% p = 0.2
Distant Disease-free Survival	58 ± 3%	55 ± 3%	57 ± 3% p = 0.6	39 ± 3%	40 ± 3% p = 0.8
Overall Survival	58 ± 3%	54 ± 3%	59 ± 3% p = 0.5	38 ± 3%	39 ± 3% p = 0.7

rXRT regional (axillary and supraclavicular) radiation therapy.

Table 1.2. Prospective randomized trials comparing total and radical mastectomy, with or without adjuvant locoregional radiotherapy

Trial	Treatment Arms	No. Patients	Followup	Results/Comments
Cancer Research Campaign[14-16]	TM vs TM + XRT^{C,A,S,I}	1140 cN− 1103 cN−	58-216 mos	No differences in survival or distant metastatic rate. XRT reduced locoregional reocurrence.
Cardiff-St. Mary's[17]	pN−: TM* vs RM pN+: TM*+XRT^A vs RM+XRT^{C,A,S,I}	75 79 49 40	− 5 years	No differences in survival rate or duration, or in distant metastatic rate.
NSABP-01[18]	RM + TSPA/placebo vs RM + XRT^{A,S,I}	633 470	5 years	No differences in survival or distant metastatic rate. XRT reduced regional nodal recur.
Oslo[19,20]	RM/OvRT vs RM/OvRT + XRT$^{A,S,I+C}$†	542 548	11-20 years	No differences in survival or distant metastatic rate. XRT reduced regional recurrences in pN+ patients.
Milan NCI[21]	RM vs RM + IMND	374 342	10 years	No differences in survival or disease-free survival.

TM	total mastectomy	XRT	radiotherapy
cN−	clinical node-negative	cN+	clinical node-positive
pN+	pathological node-positive	TSPA	triethylenethiophosphoramide
IMND	internal mammary node dissection		

RM radical mastectomy
pN− pathological node-negative
OvRT ovarian irradiation

XRT superscripts: C, chest wall; A, axillary; S, supraclavicular; I, internal mammary

* These patients also had pectoral node biopsy.
† XRT regimen changed during study; the earlier was orthovoltage/lower dose and the more recent was supervoltage/high dose.

three cN- treatment arms or between the two cN+ arms (Table 1.1). Of the cN- patients treated by radical mastectomy, 40% were found to have histological evidence of disease in their axillary lymph nodes. However, among cN- patients treated by total mastectomy alone, only 17.8% subsequently developed palpable axillary metastases. As this was a randomized trial with good balance between treatment arms in terms of patient and disease characteristics, it can be inferred with confidence that about 40% of this latter group had also harbored occult axillary disease at the time of initial treatment.

This trial provided irrefutable evidence that breast cancer mortality is not mitigated by radical surgery or locoregional radiation therapy. Patients treated by total mastectomy fared as well as those undergoing radical mastectomy. The NSABP B-04 results also laid to rest the concern that dissection of positive axillary nodes might eventuate in increased breast cancer mortality through iatrogenic dissemination of tumor cells.

NSABP B-04 further demonstrated that not all occult axillary nodal metastases become clinically significant, and that axillary metastases, while significant of a high risk of distant disease, are not causally related to systemic breast cancer metastasis. The poor predictive value of clinical axillary findings vis-á-vis nodal status was reflected in the 40% of cN- radical mastectomy patients with histologically positive nodes, and the 27% of cN+ axillae in the radical mastectomy arm in which no metastatic disease was found on histopathology.[13]

Several other prospective randomized clinical trials have also shown that neither the extent of radical surgery nor adjuvant locoregional radiotherapy (XRT) alters survival or long-term cure rates in breast cancer patients (Table 1.2). Regional nodal irradiation did result in significant reduction in recurrences within the treatment field in these trials.[14-20] In essence, these studies show that the primary therapeutic role of surgery and XRT in the management of early breast cancer relates to control of the primary tumor and regional nodal disease, and not to prevention of distant metastases. The importance of axillary nodal status as a strong predictor of prognosis and determinant for adjuvant systemic therapy is now well established. Axillary lymphadenectomy therefore has several important roles in the management of early breast cancer; accurate disease staging, triage of patients for adjuvant systemic therapy and clearance of metastatic disease from the axilla for disease control in this region (see chapter 5).

In the Milan trial of radical mastectomy with or without internal mammary node dissection (IMND),[21] the incidence of internal mammary nodal metastases in the IMND group was 20.5%. Although subsequent parasternal recurrences were therefore expected in 75 patients in the radical mastectomy (no IMND) arm, these were observed in only 15. As with axillary metastases in the NSABP B-04 trial, the risk of developing clinically significant internal mammary nodal disease is much lower than the histopathological incidence of metastasis to this lymph node chain would predict.

BREAST-CONSERVING THERAPY FOR EARLY BREAST CANCER

In 1954 Mustakallio[22] reported a series of 127 patients followed for five years or longer who had been treated for early breast cancer by local excision of the primary tumor plus postoperative orthovoltage irradiation of the breast and axilla to a dose of 2100 rad. Survival in this series was comparable to that of patients undergoing radical surgery, and the incidence of local recurrence was within acceptable limits.

Peters[23] reported a series of patients treated between 1939 and 1972 by wide local excision with or without radiotherapy, and compared these results with those observed in a matched control group treated by radical mastectomy with or without radiation. There was little difference in long term outcome between the two groups of patients. Clark et al[24-26] treated 1504 axillary node-negative patients between 1958 and 1984 by breast-conserving surgery alone or with breast radiotherapy. Again, survival compared favorably with series treated by radical surgery. However, tumor recurrence in the ipsilateral breast developed within the first ten years of followup in 29% of nonirradiated patients as compared to 14% of the irradiated group. In 94% of cases, ipsilateral breast relapses occurred within or adjacent to the site of the original primary cancer. The results of a number of other nonrandomized studies are in agreement with these findings, reporting local (breast) recurrence rates of 3.7% to 17.1% at 5 years.[27-36]

There are now seven prospective randomized clinical trials which confirm that patients undergoing breast-conserving surgery with or without radiotherapy are at no greater risk of dying of breast cancer than those

Table 1.3. Prospective randomized clinical trials comparing the efficacy of breast-conserving therapy and radical/total mastectomy in the management of early breast cancer

Trial	Treatment Arms	No. Patients	Followup	Results	Comments
Guy's Hospital[43,44]	ET + XRT[B,A,S,I] RM + XRT[A,S,I]	182 188	5-10 yrs	OS: p = NS DDFS: p = NS	Breast relapse in ET cN– patients had no effect on risk for mortality. ET: 3 cm normal breast margins. Axillary relapse rate was 22% in ET arm as nodes not removed. XRT was orthovoltage, inadequate dose by modern standards.
Milan NCI[45-47]	QUART RM	352 349	10-13 yrs	OS: p = NS DDFS: p = NS	Primary tumors < 2 cm, cN–. QUART implied resection of an entire breast quadrant, and included full axillary clearance. XRT: 50 Gy to breast + 10 Gy boost to tumor bed.
Institut Gustave-Roussy[48]	Tu/AND + XRT[B] TM/AND	88 91	10 yrs	OS: p = NS DDFS: p = NS	Primary tumors ≤ 2 cm, resected with 2 cm margins. Statistical power of trial only 50%. XRT: 45 Gy to breast + 15 Gy boost to tumor bed.
NSABP B-06[38-42]	SM/AND SM/AND + XRT[B] TM/AND	636 629 590	9 yrs	OS: p = NS DFS: p = NS DDFS: p = NS	Primary tumor ≤ 4 cm, microscopically clear surgical margins. The only three arm trial, and therefore provides the most information on breast recurrence following conservative surgery. XRT: 50 Gy to breast, no boost.
EORTC 10801[49]	SM/AND + XRT[B] TM/AND	456 426	8 yrs	OS: p = NS DDFS: p = NS	Primary tumors ≤ 5 cm, 1 cm normal breast margins. Breast relapse after SM prognostically significant. XRT: 50 Gy to breast + 25 Gy Ir[192] boost to tumor bed.
U.S. NCI[50]	SM/AND + XRT[B] TM/AND	121 116	5 yrs	OS: p = NS DDFS: p = NS	Primary tumors ≤ 5 cm; microscopically tumor-free margins not required. XRT: 48.6 Gy to breast +15–20 Gy boost.
DBCG-82TM[51]	SM/AND + XRT[B] TM/AND	430 429	6 yrs	OS: p = NS DFS: p = NS	Primary tumors of over 5 cm included. Microscopically involved margins in 27 SM/AND patients. XRT: 50 Gy to breast + 10–25 Gy boost tumor bed.

ET	extended tylectomy	OS	overall survival	DDFS	distant disease-free survival
RM	radical mastectomy	DFS	disease-free survival	p = NS	p not significant
cN–	clinical node-negative	Tu	tumorectomy	AND	axillary node dissection
TM	total mastectomy	SM	segmental mastectomy or lumpectomy		
XRT	radiotherapy	QUART	quadrantectomy, axillary clearance and breast radiotherapy		

XRT superscripts: C, chest wall; A, axillary; S, supraclavicular; I, internal mammary treated by mastectomy[37] (Table 1.3). The NSABP B-06 trial comparing total mastectomy, segmental mastectomy and segmental mastectomy plus postoperative breast radiotherapy clearly demonstrates that there is no survival advantage associated with conservative or radical breast cancer treatment, or with the use of radiation in combination with breast-conserving surgery (Table 1.4). A variety of conservative locoregional treatment regimens were compared to radical surgery in the other six trials as in NSABP B-06; no treatment-related differences in disease-specific mortality or incidence of distant metastasis were observed.

IPSILATERAL BREAST TUMOR RECURRENCE AND ADJUVANT THERAPY

RADIOTHERAPY

The NSABP B-06 trial[38-42] comparing total mastectomy (TM), segmental mastectomy (SM) and segmental mastectomy plus breast radiotherapy (SM+XRT) is especially important because it is the only three-arm study (the extra arm being conservative surgery without XRT) of breast-conserving treatment conducted to date. This trial included patients with primary lesions of up to 4 cm in diameter, and required that SM margins of resection be microscopically free of tumor involvement. As this study included patients treated by SM without XRT, the effect of XRT on local (ipsilateral breast) recurrence could be studied. Three other prospective randomized two-arm trials (conservative surgery with and without XRT) have also addressed this question (Table 1.5).

In aggregate, these studies have established beyond doubt that XRT significantly reduces the risk of ipsilateral breast tumor recurrence in patients undergoing breast-conserving surgery. All three trials required that surgical margins of resection in the breast be microscopically free of tumor. The borderline significance of the difference in local recurrence between the two groups in the Uppsala-Örebro trial[53] can probably be attributed to the limited followup time at the date of publication. In addition, the eligibility criteria for this trial (unifocal cancers no larger than 2 cm, with pathologically negative axillary nodes) were intended to include only patients at very low risk for breast tumor relapse; radiotherapy could only make a modest, perhaps statistically insignificant, improvement on the relatively low incidence of breast relapse in the nonirradiated group.

Table 1.4. Eight-year survival results of the NSABP B-06 trial[39]

	Total Mastectomy	Segmental Mastectomy With or Without bXRT	
No. Patients	590	1265*	
Disease-free Survival	58 ± 2.6%	54 ± 2.4%	p = 0.3
Distant Disease-free Survival	65 ± 2.6%	62 ± 2.3%	p = 0.4
Overall Survival	71 ± 2.6%	71 ± 2.1%	p = 0.8

* This number represents the combined total of patients in the segmental mastectomy plus radiotherapy arm (n = 629) and the segmental mastectomy only arm (n = 636). There was no difference between the two segmental mastectomy arms with respect to distant disease-free survival or overall survival.
bXRT adjuvant breast radiotherapy

Table 1.5. Prospective randomized clinical trials demonstrating the effect on ipsilateral breast tumor recurrence of radiotherapy in patients treated by breast-conserving surgery (BCS)

Trials	No. Patients			Local Recurrence Rates			Comments
	BCS	BCS + XRT	Followup	BCS	BCS + XRT		
NSABP B-06[38-42]	636	629	5 years	28%	8%	p < .001	Primary tumor size ≤ 4 cm. Included both axillary pN– and pN+ disease. Surgery consisted of segmental mastectomy with tumor-free margins on histology (no minimum gross margin).
			8 years	39%	10%	p < .001	
			9 years	43%	12%	p < .000005	
Milan NCI[52]	288	290	28-54 mos	8.8%	0.3%	p < .001	Primary tumor size ≤ 2.5 cm. Included both axillary pN– and pN+ disease. Surgery consisted of quadrantectomy with tumor-free margins on histology.
Uppsala-Örebro BCSG[53]	194	187	3 years	7.6%	2.9%	p = .06	Primary tumor size ≤ 2 cm, unifocal. Only pN– disease included. Surgery consisted of "sector resection", with histologically confirmed 20 mm tumor-free margins around the primary lesion.
Ontario Clinical Oncology Group[54]	421	416	31 mos	14.3%	2.2%	p = .0001	Primary tumor size ≤ 4 cm. Only pN– disease included. Surgery consisted of segmental mastectomy with 0.5 to 1.0 cm tumor-free margins on histology.

SYSTEMIC ADJUVANT THERAPY

NSABP B-06 node-positive patients all received postoperative adjuvant melphalan and 5-fluorouracil systemic chemotherapy. Analysis at 5 and 8 years followup unexpectedly revealed that node-positive patients in the SM+XRT arm had significantly fewer ipsilateral breast relapses than node-negative SM+XRT-treated patients, who received no chemotherapy. It was concluded that XRT and chemotherapy may be synergistic in their effects on local recurrence, and that more modern systemic adjuvant therapeutic regimens might have an even greater salutary effect on the incidence of ipsilateral breast tumor relapse.[38,39,41]

Subsequent NSABP systemic adjuvant treatment trials have been analyzed for effects of hormonal or cytotoxic chemotherapy on the incidence of local recurrence.[41] The NSABP B-13 trial, in which sequential methotrexate and 5-fluorouracil/leukovorin was compared to no chemotherapy in node-negative estrogen receptor-negative breast cancer patients, demonstrated a 67% reduction in breast relapses in the chemotherapy arm at 54 months. In the most recent analysis of the NSABP B-14 results (five years followup),[55] 4.4% of patients in the placebo arm had developed ipsilateral breast tumor recurrence as compared to 1.5% of tamoxifen-treated patients (p < 0.00001).

In node-positive receptor-negative patients in the NSABP B-15 study, local recurrence was less frequent in the arm treated with concurrent CMF chemotherapy and

XRT (2.9%) as compared to the other two groups in which XRT was administered only after completion of doxorubicin-based cytotoxic therapy (5.7% and 6.0% local recurrence). In node-positive receptor-positive patients treated with either tamoxifen or tamoxifen plus doxorubicin-based chemotherapy, local recurrence was very infrequent (only one breast failure among all 232 patients at 44 months), as previously observed in the B-06 trial.[41]

The rate of ipsilateral breast relapse per year in B-06 node-negative receptor-positive patients (to whom no chemotherapy was administered) was the same as that in the untreated B-14 arm (1.2%). Similarly, in node-negative receptor-negative B-06 and B-13 patients who received no adjuvant chemotherapy, yearly local recurrence rates were 2.2% and 2.3% respectively. However, in the chemotherapy arm of B-13 and the tamoxifen arm of B-14, the yearly rates of ipsilateral breast recurrence were only 0.7% and 0.5%. This comparison of systemic therapy-related effects on breast failures was made at a similar time at risk for all three trials (Fig. 1.1).

Similar observations have been made elsewhere. Solin et al[56] at the University of Pennsylvania reported local recurrences in 3% of node-positive patients treated by breast-conserving surgery, radiotherapy and chemotherapy as compared to 8% among patients treated by surgery plus irradiation only. Rose et al[57] at the Joint Center for Radiation Therapy compared 74 chemotherapy plus breast conservation-treated patients to 192 patients treated with breast-conserving therapy only. Despite the fact that the former group had higher T and N stage tumors, only 4% had their initial recurrence in the breast as compared to 15% of those who did not receive chemotherapy. Haffty et al[58] compared the incidence of local recurrence in pathological node-positive patients, 88% of whom received adjuvant cyclophosphamide, methotrexate and 5-fluorouracil chemotherapy or tamoxifen, to that of node-negative patients of whom only 8% were treated with adjuvant systemic therapy. Despite their higher stage of disease, local recurrence developed in only 6% of Stage II patients as compared to 13% of those with Stage I disease (p = 0.08).

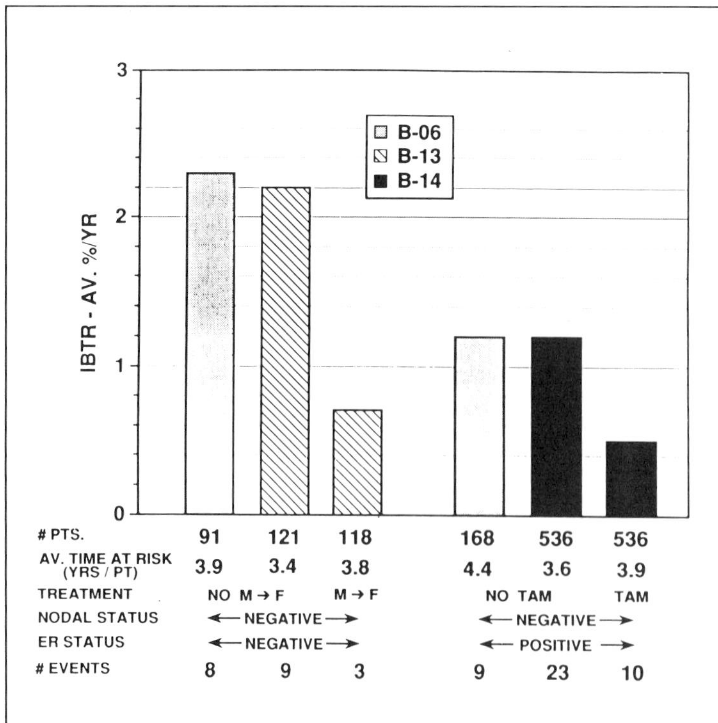

Fig. 1.1. Ipsilateral breast tumor recurrence per year following segmental mastectomy with postoperative ipsilateral breast irradiation. This shows the relationship of breast recurrence to nodal status, estrogen receptor (ER) status and postoperative adjuvant systemic therapy in the NSABP B-06, B-13 and B-14 trials. Reproduced with permission from Wiley–Liss, a Division of John Wiley and Sons, Inc., Fisher B, et al. Semin Surg Oncol 1992; 8:153-160; © 1992.

Thus, adjuvant systemic therapy appears to mitigate the risk of ipsilateral breast tumor recurrence in patients undergoing breast-conserving therapy.

CURRENT STATUS OF BREAST-CONSERVING TREATMENT

Debate continues on many issues pertaining to optimization of breast conservation therapy for early breast cancer. These will be discussed in further detail in chapters 2 to 4. There is no longer any doubt, however, that radical cancer surgery offers no survival advantage over conservative locoregional treatment.

There is a prodigious and rapidly expanding literature on the results of breast-conserving treatment in patients with early breast cancer. Regimens in use worldwide employ surgery and radiotherapy in various combinations and permutations. Some require more extensive breast resections (quadrantectomy or partial mastectomy) or microscopically tumor-free margins of resection, while in others excision of gross disease is considered adequate irrespective of the histopathological status of surgical margins (Table 1.3). Similarly, there are variations in radiation techniques in terms of dosage, irradiation fields (breast versus breast and regional lymphatics) and the use of external beam or interstitial boosts to the primary tumor site in the breast. NSABP protocols specify only irradiation of the conserved breast to 50 Gy with no boost,[59] whereas other groups boost the tumor bed dosage by an additional 10 to 20 Gy.[60,61] The specifics of breast-conserving surgery and adjuvant breast radiotherapy will be addressed in greater detail in the next chapter.

In general, the more limited in scope the breast surgery, the more aggressive the radiotherapeutic approach, and vice versa.[62] There is similar diversity in the management of the axillary lymph nodes (see chapter 5). The American College of Surgery, the American College of Radiology, the College of American Pathologists and the Society of Surgical Oncology have recently compiled a report in which these variations have been addressed and, where possible, reconciled in

a useful summation of the principles of breast-conserving therapy.[37]

SURGEONS, PATIENTS AND TREATMENT DECISIONS

There is concern in some quarters that breast-conserving therapy is not being offered to patients or practiced as much as it should be. In an analysis of breast cancer cases in the Colorado Central Cancer Registry, Tarbox et al[63] found that 72% of patients with T1 primary breast cancers registered within the preceding five years had been treated by modified radical mastectomy. In their survey of the beliefs and practice patterns of 123 surgeons who performed breast cancer surgery, 27 respondents professed the belief that breast-conserving surgery is inferior to mastectomy in terms of survival while 54 believed the two operations to be equivalent. The former cohort of surgeons performed breast-conserving operations 36% and total mastectomy 64% of the time for T1 breast cancer. The second group performed conservative surgery in 55% and mastectomy in 45% of such patients. The remaining 42 surgeons believed the two options were equivalent but felt that modified radical mastectomy was the gold standard and the cosmetic outcome of breast conservation was frequently compromised by the use of postoperative radiotherapy. They therefore biased their presentation of the treatment options to patients in favor of mastectomy. This group of surgeons performed segmental mastectomy in 40% and total mastectomy in 60% of patients.

When asked why patients tend to choose modified radical mastectomy more often than might be expected, a majority of respondent surgeons noted that some patients need to feel that "everything has been done", and others are dissuaded by fear or the inconvenience of five to six weeks of radiotherapy.[63]

These findings did not fully explain the preponderance of mastectomy-treated patients in the Cancer Registry. Tarbox et al[63] postulated that surgeons may unconsciously bias their preoperative treatment discussions with patients in favor of total mastectomy. Other studies have also suggested persistent reluctance of some surgeons to accept the equivalent efficacy of conservative therapy and mastectomy in early breast cancer. There may be a need for ongoing education of professionals in community practice on this issue, and on the importance of taking the time to discuss treatment options for early breast cancer in as objective a manner as possible.

While there is merit in this criticism, it would be simplistic to suggest that medical professionals are solely or even primarily responsible for the fact that a substantial proportion of breast cancer patients eligible for breast conservation still undergo modified radical mastectomy. Even among surveyed healthy women given an informed choice between the two options in the hypothetical event of being diagnosed with early breast carcinoma, only 49% of respondents chose breast-conserving therapy.[64,65] The reasons why breast cancer patients make certain treatment decisions after complete, objective disclosure of relevant information are subtle and complex. It was once anticipated that patients treated conservatively would suffer less psychosocial morbidity than mastectomized patients, but this benefit has not been as clear-cut as anticipated. A discussion of recent data pertinent to these issues follows.

Locoregional breast cancer therapy, either conservative or radical, precipitates major sexual dysfunction, marital breakdown or psychological problems in perhaps 25% of patients. Many or most affected individuals have preexisting psychosexual, psychological or marital difficulties.[66,67] The strongest predictors of postoperative emotional morbidity are the patient's overall psychological health, stability and satisfaction in a marital relationship, and premorbid sex life. In careful studies of patients treated by breast conservation and those who had modified radical mastectomy, there were no significant treatment-related differences in quality of life, performance status, psychological adjustment, mood disturbance or marital happiness.[66-71] Of the studies which evaluated the effects of breast cancer surgery on sexual frequency or satisfaction, the only one reporting a positive result was the prospective analysis of Pozo et al,[71] which showed a difference in

favor of breast conservation at six and twelve months post surgery.

Interestingly, systemic adjuvant chemotherapy has the strongest negative impact on sexuality because of the induced ovarian failure. Premature menopause and decreased sexual desire and arousability related to loss of ovarian androgens are significant problems in patients requiring postoperative cytotoxic therapy.[66]

Not surprisingly, patients treated by breast-conserving treatment have a more positive body image postoperatively than those undergoing total mastectomy.[66-68] Mastectomy-treated women report distressing limitations in clothing selection, difficulties with mastectomy prostheses, increased discomfiture with nudity especially in the presence of others, and anxiety about their sexual desirability.[66,67,72] Breast reconstruction has a salutary effect on all of these concerns; this benefit does not seem to be affected by the timing (immediate versus delayed) of reconstructive surgery.[66,67] Women having breast reconstruction report that the procedure contributes to their feeling whole again, allows much more discretion in choice of clothing and eliminates the problems attendant with a breast prosthesis.

Fear of disease recurrence might be expected to be higher in patients undergoing breast-conserving treatment. However, the data on this question are confusing and contradictory. On balance, fear of recurrence is most prevalent among those requiring completion mastectomy for local recurrence following breast-conserving surgery, patients with positive nodes, patients who undergo adjuvant chemotherapy, and those with preexisting psychological fragility.[67,73]

Having to confront a diagnosis of breast cancer is an emotionally traumatic experience for any woman. However, there is no question that breast cancer patients are perfectly capable of making rational treatment choices when given all of the medically relevant information.[70] Indeed, active participation of the patient in treatment decisions may expedite her psychologically coming to terms with the disease and treatment sequelae.[67,70] The particular treatment chosen by the individual is less important to her psychological well-being than the preoperative efforts of her surgeon to make her a well informed patient, aware of all the options as well as the benefits and risks of each. Once apprised of the facts, and in spite of strong encouragement by their surgeons to opt for less radical treatment, a proportion of breast cancer patients may freely choose not to have conservative treatment. For example, of 216 candidates for conservative surgery counseled by Wolberg,[70] only 103 chose to save the affected breast. Patients choosing total mastectomy cite a desire for rapid completion of treatment, fear of future cancers, and reluctance to have radiation postoperatively as the reasons for their decision. Those who opt for breast conservation place a higher value on saving the breast, and may have less fear of recurrence.[70,73,74] In the final analysis, the sexual and aesthetic consequences of breast cancer surgery are balanced or even overshadowed by concerns about breast cancer mortality in the minds of many patients. A high prevalence of concern about breast cancer recurrence and future health among breast cancer patients studied 2 to 11 years postoperatively was documented by Sneeuw et al.[75] Pozo et al[71] suggested that this important factor may have been given insufficient weight in most published analyses of the psychosexual effects of cancer treatment.

Not all women wish to make their own choice, and a few may even request that the physician or surgeon take the initiative in this regard. When medical factors suggest that either segmental or total mastectomy would be satisfactory, it is appropriate and desirable that medical professionals encourage the patient in the direction of breast conservation. However, breast cancer patients retain the prerogative to exercise their own judgement in treatment selection. Each woman has a unique perspective on the disease and its treatment, and has her own emotional needs and aspirations for herself and her family. Given that breast conservation and mastectomy have equal efficacy in early breast cancer, and that there are few differences between them in terms of psy-

chological sequelae, treatment discussions should be thorough and recommendations should take into account the individual patient's concerns about quality of life.

Perhaps the most significant benefit of the advent of breast conserving therapy is that it offers so many breast cancer patients a choice where none previously existed. This does not necessarily mean that all women will be more comfortable with this option than traditional mastectomy with or without reconstruction.

REFERENCES

1. Robinson JO. Treatment of breast cancer through the ages. Amer J Surg 1986; 151:317-332

2. Kardinal CG, Yarbro JW. A conceptual history of cancer. Semin Oncol 1979; 6:396-408.

3. Moffat FL, Ketcham AS. Surgery for malignant neoplasia. The evolution of on-cological surgery and its role in the management of cancer. In: McKenna RJ Sr., Murphy GL, eds. Cancer Surgery. Philadelphia: JB Lippincott 1994; 1-20.

4. Robertson HR. Without benefit of anaesthesia: George Wilson's amputation and Fanny Burney's mastectomy. Ann Roy Coll Phys Surg Canada 1989; 22:27-30.

5. Halsted WS. The results of radical operations for the cure of cancer of the breast. Ann Surg 1907; 46:1-19.

6. Sugarbaker ED. Extended radical mastectomy. Its superiority in the treatment of breast cancer. J Amer Med Asoc 1964; 187: 96-99.

7. Veronesi U, Zingo L. Extended radical mastectomy for cancer of the breast. Cancer 1967; 20:677-680.

8. Urban JA, Baker HW. Radical mastectomy in continuity with en bloc resection of the internal mammary lymph chain. Cancer 1952; 5:992-1008.

9. Patey DH, Dyson WH. The prognosis of carcinoma of the breast in relation to the type of operation performed. Br J Cancer 1948; 2:7-13.

10. Patey DH. A review of 146 cases of carcinoma of the breast operated on between 1930 and 1943. Br J Cancer 1967; 21: 260-269.

11. McWhirter R. The value of a simple mastectomy and radiotherapy in the treatment of cancer of the breast. Br J Radiol 1948; 21:599-610.

12. McWhirter R. Should more radical treatment be attempted in breast cancer? Amer J Roentgenol 1964; 92:3-13.

13. Fisher B, Redmond C, Fisher ER, et al. Ten-year results of a randomized clinical trial comparing radical mastectomy and total mastectomy with or without radiation. New Engl J Med 1985; 312:674-681.

14. Cancer Research Campaign Working Party. Cancer Research Campaign (King's/ Cambridge) trial for early breast cancer. Lancet 1980; 1:55-60.

15. Berstock DA, Houghton J, Haybittle J, Baum M. The role of radiotherapy following total mastectomy for patients with early breast cancer. World J Surg 1985; 9:667-670.

16. Haybittle JL, Brinkley D, Houghton J, A'Hern RP, Baum M. Postoperative radiotherapy and late mortality: evidence from the Cancer Research Campaign trial for early breast cancer. Br Med J 1989; 298:16 11-1614.

17. Forrest APM, Roberts MM, Cant ELM, et al. Simple mastectomy and pectoral node biopsy: the Cardiff-St. Mary's trial. World J Surg 1977; 1:320-323.

18. Fisher B, Slack NH, Cavanaugh PJ, et al. Postoperative radiotherapy in the treatment of breast cancer. Ann Surg 1970; 172: 711-732.

19. Høst H, Brennhovd IO. The effect of postoperative radiotherapy in breast cancer. Int J Radiat Oncol Biol Phys 1977; 2: 1061-1067.

20. Høst H, Brennhovd IO, Loeb M. Postoperative radiotherapy in breast cancer - long-term results from the Oslo study. Int J Radiat Oncol Biol Phys 1986; 12:727-732.

21. Veronesi U, Valagussa P. Inefficacy of internal mammary node dissection in breast cancer surgery. Cancer 1981; 47:170-173.

22. Mustakallio S. Treatment of breast cancer by tumour extirpation and roentgen therapy instead of radical operation. J Fac Radiol 1954; 6:23-26.

23. Peters MV. Wedge resection with or without radiation in early breast cancer. Int J Radiat Oncol Biol Phys 1977; 2:1151-1156.

24. Clark RM, Wilkinson RH, Mahoney LJ, Reid JG, MacDonald WD. Breast cancer: a 21 year experience with conservative surgery and radiation. Int J Radiat Oncol Biol Phys 1982; 8:967-975.

25. Clark RM, Wilkinson RH, Mahoney LJ, Reid JG, MacDonald WD. Breast cancer: a 22 year study of the conservative approach. Rev Endocrine-Related Cancer 1984; Suppl 4:227-232.

26. Clark RM, Wilkinson RH, Miceli PN, MacDonald WD. Breast cancer. Experiences with conservation therapy. Amer J Clin Oncol 1987; 10:461-468.

27. Calle R, Pilleron JP, Schlienger P, Vilcoq JR. Conservative management of operable breast cancer. Ten years' experience at the Foundation Curie. Cancer 1978; 42: 2045-2053.

28. Hellman S, Harris JR, Levene MB. Radiation therapy of early carcinoma of the breast without mastectomy. Cancer 1980; 46:988-994.

29. Crile G Jr. Results of conservative treatment of breast cancer at ten and 15 years. Ann Surg 1975; 181:26-30.

30. Hermann RE, Esselstyn CB, Crile G, Cooperman AM, Antunez AR, Hoerr SI. Results of conservative operations for breast cancer. Arch Surg 1985; 120:746-751.

31. Montague ED, Gutierrez AE, Barker JL, Tapley N duV, Fletcher GH. Conservation surgery and irradiation for the treatment of favorable breast cancer. Cancer 1979; 43:1058-1061.

32. Montague ED, Fletcher GH. The curative value of irradiation in the treatment of nondisseminated breast cancer. Cancer 1980; 46:995-998.

33. Chu AM, Cope O, Russo R, et al. Treatment of early stage breast cancer by limited surgery and radical irradiation. Int J Radiat Oncol Biol Phys 1980; 6:25-30.

34. Pierquin B, Owen R, Maylin C, et al. Radical radiation therapy of breast cancer. Int J Radiat Oncol Biol Phys 1980; 6:17-24.

35. Poisson R, Legault-Poisson S, Mercier J-P. Pilot study of the individualized non-mutilating treatment of breast cancer (personal experience from 1970 to 1976). Rev Endocrine-Related Cancer 1984; suppl 4:223-226.

36. Prosnitz LR, Goldenberg IS, Packard RA, et al. Radiation therapy as initial treatment for early stage cancer of the breast without mastectomy. Cancer 1977; 39:917-923.

37. Winchester DP, Cox JD. Standards for breast conservation treatment. CA - A Cancer Journal for Clinicians 1992; 42:134-162.

38. Fisher B, Bauer M, Margolese R, et al. Five-year results of a randomized clinical trial comparing total mastectomy and segmental mastectomy with or without radiation in the treatment of breast cancer. New Engl J Med 1985; 312:665-673.

39. Fisher B, Redmond C, Poisson R, et al. Eight-year results of a randomized clinical trial comparing total mastectomy and lumpectomy with or without irradiation in the treatment of breast cancer. New Engl J Med 1989; 320:822-828.

40. Fisher B, Anderson S, Fisher ER, et al. Significance of ipsilateral breast tumor recurrence after lumpectomy. Lancet 1992; 338:327-331.

41. Fisher B, Wickerham DL, Deutsch M, Anderson S, Redmond C, Fisher ER. Breast tumor recurrence following lumpectomy with or without breast irradiation: an overview of recent NSABP findings. Semin Surg Oncol 1992; 8:153-160.

42. Fisher B, Redmond C, and NSABP authors. Lumpectomy for breast cancer: an update of the NSABP experience. J Natl Cancer Inst Monogr 1992; 11:7-13.

43. Atkins H, Hayward JL, Klugman DJ, Wayte AB. Treatment of early breast cancer: a report after ten years of a clinical trial. Br Med J 1972; 2:423-429.

44. Hayward JL. The Guy's trial of treatments of "early" breast cancer. World J Surg 1977; 1:314-316.

45. Veronesi U, Banfi A, Del Vecchio M, et al. Comparison of Halsted mastectomy with quadrantectomy, axillary dissection and radiotherapy in early breast cancer: long-term results. Eur J Cancer Clin Oncol 1986; 22:1085-1089.

46. Veronesi U, Banfi A, Salvadori B, et al. Breast conservation is the treatment of choice in small breast cancer: long-term results of a randomized trial. Eur J Cancer Clin Oncol 1990; 26:668-670.

47. Veronesi U, Saccozzi R, Del Vecchio M, et al. Comparing radical mastectomy with quadrantectomy, axillary dissection and radiotherapy in patients with small cancers of the breast. New Engl J Med 1981; 305:6-11.

48. Sarrazin D, Le MG, Arriagada R, et al. Ten-year results of a randomized trial comparing a conservative treatment to mastectomy in early breast cancer. Radiother Oncol 1989; 14:177-184.

49. van Dongen JA, Bartelink H, Fentiman IS, et al. Randomized clinical trial to assess the value of breast-conserving therapy in Stage I and II breast cancer, EORTC 10801 trial. J Natl Cancer Inst Monogr 1992; 11:15-18.

50. Straus K, Lichter A, Lippman M, et al. Results of the National Cancer Institute early breast cancer trial. J Natl Cancer Inst Monogr 1992; 11:27-32.

51. Blichert-Toft M, Rose C, Andersen JA, et al. Danish randomized trial comparing breast conservation therapy with mastectomy: six years of life-table analysis. J Natl Cancer Inst Monogr 1992; 11:19-25.

52. Veronesi U, Luini A, Del Vecchio M, et al. Radiotherapy after breast-preserving surgery in women with localized cancer of the breast. New Engl J Med 1993; 328:1587-1591.

53. Uppsala-Örebro Breast Cancer Study Group. Sector resection with or without postoperative radiotherapy for Stage I breast cancer: a randomized trial. J Natl Cancer Inst 1990; 82:277-282.

54. Clark R, McCulloch P, Levine M, Lipa M, Wilkinson R. A randomized clinical trial to assess the effectiveness of breast irradiation following lumpectomy and axillary dissection for node-negative breast cancer. Proc Amer Soc Clin Oncol 1990; 9:21 (Abstr).

55. Fisher B, Costantino J, Wickerham L, et al. Adjuvant therapy for node-negative breast cancer: an update of NSABP findings. Proc Amer Soc Clin Oncol 1993; 12:69 (Abstr).

56. Solin LJ, Fowble B, Martz KL, Goodman RL. Definitive irradiation for early stage breast cancer: the University of Pennsylvania experience. Int J Radiat Oncol Biol Phys 1988; 14:235-242.

57. Rose MA, Henderson IC, Gelman R, et al. Premenopausal breast cancer patients treated with conservative surgery, radiotherapy and adjuvant chemotherapy have a low risk of local failure. Int J Radiat Oncol Biol Phys 1989; 17:711-717.

58. Haffty BG, Fischer D, Rose M, Beinfield M, McKhann C. Prognostic factors for local recurrence in the conservatively treated breast cancer patient: a cautious interpretation of the data. J Clin Oncol 1991; 9: 997-1003.

59. Deutsch M. Radiotherapy after breast-conservation therapy: how much is enough? Semin Surg Oncol 1992; 8:140-146.

60. Pierce SM, Harris JR. The role of radiation therapy in the management of primary breast cancer. CA - A Cancer Journal for Clinicians 1991; 41:85-96.

61. Kurtz JM. Radiation therapy and breast preservation: past achievements, current results, and future prospects. Semin Surg Oncol 1992; 8:147-152.

62. Kinne DW. The surgical management of primary breast cancer. CA - A Cancer Journal for Clinicians 1991; 41:71-84.

63. Tarbox BB, Rockwood JK, Abernathy CM. Are modified radical mastectomies done for T1 breast cancers because of surgeon's advice or patient's choice? Amer J Surg 1992; 164:417-422.

64. Ward S, Heidrich S, Wolberg W. Factors women take into account when deciding upon type of surgery for breast cancer. Cancer Nurs 1989; 12: 344-351.

65. Wolberg W, Tanner M, Romaas E, Trump D, Malec J. Factors influencing options in primary breast cancer treatment. J Clin Oncol 1987; 5: 68-74.

66. Schover LR. The impact of breast cancer on sexuality, body image, and intimate relationships. CA - A Cancer Journal for Clinicians 1991; 41:112-120.

67. Schain WS, Fetting JH. Modified radical mastectomy versus breast conservation: psychosocial considerations. Semin Oncol 1992; 19:239-243.

68. Ganz PA, Coscarelli Schag CA, Lee J, Polinsky ML, Tan S-J. Breast conservation versus mastectomy. Is there a difference in psychological adjustment or quality of life in the year after surgery? Cancer 1992; 69:1729-1738.

69. Blichert-Toft M. Breast-conserving therapy for mammary carcinoma: psychosocial aspects, indications and limitations. Ann Med 1992; 24:445-451.

70. Wolberg WH. Mastectomy or breast conservation in the management of primary breast cancer. Oncology 1990; 4:101-104.

71. Pozo C, Carver CS, Noriega V, et al. Effects of mastectomy versus lumpectomy on emotional adjustment to breast cancer: a prospective study of the first year postsurgery. J Clin Oncol 1992; 10:1292-1298.

72. Bartelink H, van Dam F, van Dongen J. Psychological effects of breast conserving therapy in comparison with radical mastectomy. Int J Radiat Oncol Biol Phys 1985; 11:381-385.

73. Lasry J-CM, Margolese RG. Fear of recurrence, breast-conserving surgery, and the trade-off hypothesis. Cancer 1992; 69: 2111-2115.

74. Wilson RG, Hart A, Dawes PJDK. Mastectomy or conservation: the patient's choice. Br Med J 1988; 297:1167-1169.

75. Sneeuw KCA, Aaronson NK, Yarnold JR, et al. Cosmetic and functional outcomes of breast conserving treatment for early breast cancer. 2. Relationship with psychosocial functioning. Radiother Oncol 1992; 25: 160-166.

CHAPTER 2

Conservative Treatment of Invasive Breast Cancer
Surgical and Radiotherapeutic Considerations

In the preceeding chapter, the efficacy of breast-conserving treatment as compared to radical surgery was discussed. A closer look at published studies reveals that the term "breast-conserving therapy" encompasses many regimens in which surgery and radiotherapy are employed in different combinations. There are substantial variations between institutions and nations, and between North American and European centers, in what is considered optimal conservative locoregional treatment for early breast cancer. The various factors which influence the extent of surgery and type of radiation therapy will be addressed in this chapter. Potential long-term sequelae of breast-conserving therapy will also be reviewed.

SURGICAL CONSIDERATIONS

Breast-conserving operations have been given many names over the past 30 years. Only a very few of these can be considered true synonyms, and therefore considerable caution is required when using them.

The extended tylectomy in the Guy's Hospital trial[1] was defined as resection of the tumor mass plus the surrounding breast tissue within 3 cm of visible or palpable cancer. While the microscopic status of the surgical margins was not emphasized in this trial, present-day breast surgeons would concur that many if not most cancers of 4 cm or less in diameter removed in such an operation would likely have tumor-free margins on histology.

The quadrantectomy of Veronesi et al[2] encompasses approximately one-quarter of the tissue of the breast, as the name implies. The overlying skin and the pectoralis fascia are resected en bloc with the breast parenchyma. As this operation is performed for breast cancers of only 2 cm or less, it is likely that the surgical margins were free of tumor in most cases, although again this was not stipulated. A similar but more limited breast-conserving procedure, "sector resection", was used in the Uppsala-Örebro trial[3] for tumors of no more than 2 cm in size. A generous wedge or sector of breast tissue around the tumor, including pectoralis major fascia is removed; in this operation, the surgical margins are required to be histologically free of tumor involvement.

The partial mastectomy employed by Crile and colleagues at the Cleveland Clinic for tumors of 4 cm or less involved en bloc resection of the tumor and surrounding breast parenchyma with a narrow ellipse of skin encompassing the biopsy scar.[4-7] Skin flaps are undermined on either side of the ellipse in the subcutaneous plane for 1 to 2 cm beyond the edge of the biopsy cavity or palpable residual tumor, and dissection then taken down through the pectoralis major fascia (which is taken as the deep margin), staying clear of any palpable disease. The specimen is oriented and submitted for gross measurement of margins and histo-pathological examination of representative frozen sections from the inked margins. Total mastectomy is performed if histologically clear margins cannot be obtained or if the extent of resection necessary to get clear of all primary disease would leave a cosmetically unacceptable breast.

Segmental mastectomy, conceptually similar to but not synonymous with sector resection, is considered interchangeable with the term lumpectomy in NSABP parlance.[8,9] The NSABP defined segmental mastectomy and lumpectomy as resection of the carcinoma with enough surrounding normal breast tissue to yield microscopically tumor-free surgical margins. There was no minimum specified margin of breast tissue around the lesion; tumor cells could approach to within one cell's breadth of the surgical margin as long as they were not in contact with or transgressing the inked edges of the specimen. Furthermore, it was not considered necessary for the pectoralis fascia or any overlying skin (unless there was a biopsy scar, in which case this was resected en bloc) to be included in the surgical specimen. Whenever possible, development of skin flaps by undermining in the subcutaneous plane was avoided because of possible adverse effects on cosmesis.

Partial mastectomy, segmental mastectomy, lumpectomy and "sector resection" spare more of the normal breast parenchyma than quadrantectomy and are therefore cosmetically advantageous. The conservatism of these surgical operations makes histopatho-logical confirmation of tumor-free surgical margins necessary for assurance of complete tumor excision. Quadrantectomy and extended tylectomy are highly likely to yield clear margins by virtue of their extent, which lessens the need for microscopic confirmation of the margins. However, there is a greater likelihood of distortion, nipple deviation, and significant asymmetry as compared to the contralateral breast in patients undergoing these more aggressive procedures.

"Wide excision", "gross tumor excision" and "tumorectomy" are terms generally reserved for even more conservative breast operations in which only visible or palpable cancer is completely removed with a small margin of grossly normal breast tissue. No formal attempt is made to obtain histopathologically clear surgical margins. Unfortunately, such procedures have been referred to as lumpectomies on occasion;[10-13] the discrepancy between this definition and that of the NSABP adds an element of confusion whenever the term lumpectomy is used to describe a breast-conserving operation. The European Organization for Research and Treatment of Cancer,[12] the U.S. National Cancer Institute,[10,11] the Joint Center for Radiation Therapy at the Harvard Medical School,[14] the Danish Breast Cancer Collaborative Group[15,16] and various European institutions[17-21] employ surgical procedures which are limited to clearance of gross tumor only. These centers use relatively aggressive radiotherapy regimes, usually boosting the radiation dose to the tumor bed with external beam therapy or an interstitial implant.

MARGINS OF RESECTION

It has long been a tenet of oncological surgery that clinical outcome is critically dependent on complete removal of all cancer with a tumor-free margin of normal surrounding tissue. The extent of excision required may vary between types of cancer, but the principle of complete surgical clearance of tumor has historically been uniformly applied. There is general agreement that at the very least, complete excision of gross disease is most important for a successful outcome with conservative management of early breast carcinoma. However, as noted in chapter 1, some centers are less particular about the microscopic status of the surgical margins, relying instead on adjuvant radiation for prevention of local treatment failure.

At a minimum, excision of all gross tumor in the breast is necessary for adequate control of local disease by breast-conserving therapy.[19,20,22-24] "Tumorectomy" with a narrow margin of normal breast tissue both debulks the primary disease and extirpates the comparatively hypoxic, and therefore radioresistant, central core of the lesion. Other factors being equal, gross involvement of surgical margins by breast cancer implies a four- to five-fold increase in risk of tumor relapse in the primary site.[22,24] In series in which either less-than-complete gross excision of cancer or no excision was performed (usually for larger T2 tumors), acceptable local control rates were attained only by resorting to more radical radiation therapy.[19,21,23,25] Secondary surgical intervention for persistent primary or axillary disease after completion of radical radiotherapy is necessary in up to 48% of patients with large cancers when complete excision of gross tumor is either not possible or not stipulated in the breast conservation protocol.[23]

The risk of local recurrence is inversely proportional to the extent of surgical resection in patients undergoing breast-conserving surgery. Veronesi et al[13] in a prospective randomized trial compared their quadrantectomy operation to a "tumorectomy" incorporating only a 1 cm margin of grossly normal breast tissue in patients with cancers of 2.5 cm or less in greatest dimension. Both arms were treated with postoperative breast irradiation to a total dose to the tumor bed of 60 gray (Gy); the quadrantectomy patients received whole breast irradiation by Cobalt-60 or megavoltage therapy to 50 Gy over 5 weeks followed by a 10 Gy ortho-voltage boost to the tumor bed, whereas tumorectomy patients received 45 Gy over 5 weeks to the breast with a 15 Gy interstitial Iridium-192 (^{192}Ir) boost to the tumor site. At the time of publication, 24 of 345 tumorectomy patients (7.4%) and 8 of 360

quadrantectomy patients (2.2%) had developed local recurrences (p = 0.005). Among 283 tumorectomy patients in whom resection margins were evaluated histologically, recurrences developed in 6 of 46 patients (13%) with positive margins as compared to 13 recurrences among the 237 patients (5.5%) with microscopically clear margins (p = 0.12).

Vicini et al[26] analyzed the incidence of local recurrence by volume of breast tissue resected in breast-preserving operations; histopathological assessment of tumor margins was not performed. Among T1 breast cancers, the incidence of ipsilateral breast relapse was significantly reduced by excision of larger volumes of breast tissue; for T2 cancers, this was true only in those with extensive associated intraductal carcinoma. Overall, the local failure rate among lesions with extensive associated intraductal disease was greater than that of cancers in which there was little or no intraductal component (vide infra).

Recht et al[22] compared the incidence of local recurrence following complete and incomplete gross tumor excision in a retrospective analysis. Eight of 24 patients (33%) with grossly incomplete tumor excision experienced failure as compared to 22 of 342 patients (6.4%) who underwent complete resection of gross tumor (p < 0.0001 by comparison of five-year estimates of local failure rates).

Ghossein et al[27] similarly noted a significant difference in local recurrence among 323 patients undergoing gross tumorectomies, 142 patients treated by "wide excision" with 2-cm gross margins around the tumor, and 56 patients having quadrantectomy. The incidence of microscopically positive margins in each of the three groups was 41%, 14% and 7% (p < 0.001) and local recurrence eventuated in 15%, 7% and 5%, respectively (p < 0.03).

Thus, it is clear that with breast-conserving surgery, complete removal of all gross cancer is very important for optimal control of disease in the affected breast. The findings in two of these studies[13,27] further suggest that histopathological confirmation of tumor-free margins may result in even greater reduction in the risk of subsequent ipsilateral breast tumor recurrence.

There is little agreement among pathologists and surgeons on what constitutes the optimal histopathological method of assessing surgical margins.[28-30] The NSABP method[31] and variations on it are widely used today in North America. This technique is a useful reference point in discussions of surgical margin assessment because of the extensive experience with the method and verification of its utility in the NSABP clinical trials. It is relatively easy to follow, and relies on both gross and histopathological evaluation of the segmental mastectomy (Fig. 2.1).

The NSABP segmental mastectomy or lumpectomy requires that the surgeon resect the primary tumor with enough surrounding normal breast tissue to accomplish complete excision of all gross tumor with microscopic verification of tumor-free margins. Once removed, the segmental mastectomy specimen is properly oriented with sutures marking particular margins (superior, lateral, deep, etc.) and immediately submitted to the pathologist in the fresh state. Ideally, the surgeon should then take additional samples of suspicious, firm, fibrous or other nonfatty tissue from the superior, inferior, medial, lateral and deep margins of the surgical defect in the breast and submit them separately for intraoperative histopathological confirmation of clear margins.[31]

Prior to cutting the breast specimen, the pathologist paints the entire exterior surface with India ink or a comparable dye. The margins are then assessed grossly by incising the segmental mastectomy through appropriate planes, and the surgeon is informed of any surgical margins close to or involved by gross disease. The surgeon may then take an additional margin of tissue from the corresponding parenchymal surface

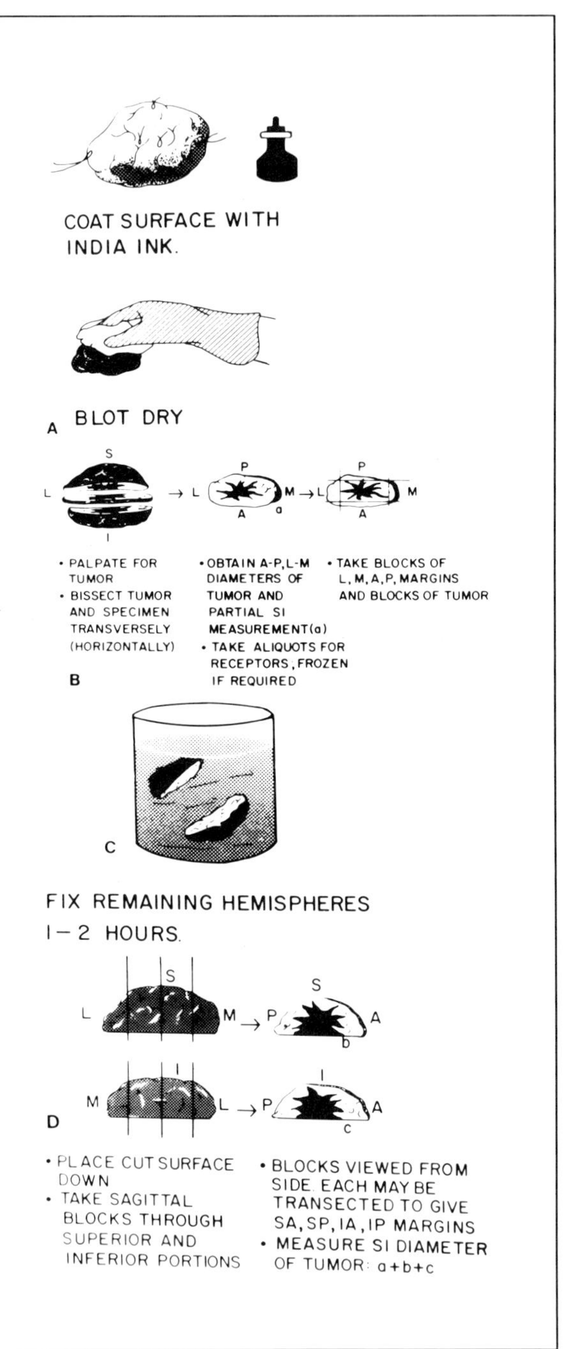

Fig. 2.1. The method of gross and histopathological assessment recommended by the NSABP. Reproduced with permission from Fisher B, et al. World J Surg 1985; 9:692-698.

in the surgical wound and mark the new margin in the re-excision specimen with ink or a suture. This is then frozen for microscopic verification of tumor clearance.

The inked margins of the segmental mastectomy specimens were involved by tumor in 10% of patients randomized to the breast conservation arms in the NSABP B-06 trial, mandating completion mastectomy as stipulated in the study protocol. Surgical margins were involved in 15% of those with positive axillary nodes as compared to 7% of node-negative patients, and the incidence of positive margins increased with the number of involved lymph nodes. Patients whose primary tumors ranged in size from 2.1 to 4.0 cm were more likely to have margin involvement by tumor than those with smaller cancers (13% versus 7%). Positive margins were seen most frequently in patients with centrally situated cancers.[8]

McCormick et al[32] reported 108 patients treated by breast conservation at Memorial Hospital in whom the margins of resection were assessed microscopically by a method similar to that used by NSABP investigators. Of the 75 patients in whom the initial excision was performed by Memorial Hospital surgeons, 28% were found to have microscopically positive margins; the extent of involvement usually was limited to focal extension of tumor to one margin only. The incidence of positive surgical margins increased with tumor size but was not influenced by nodal status in this series.

The importance of microscopically tumor-free surgical margins for optimal results in breast-conserving therapy is not universally acknowledged. The NSABP and its participating institutions consider histopathologically negative margins to be an essential prerequisite for acceptable local control rates with breast-conserving therapy.

Retrospective analyses from a number of centers[27,33-39] support the stance of the NSABP on this issue, while other authors have suggested that the microscopic status of margins may not be critical for control of disease in the breast.[40-44] It is noteworthy that in at least three of these latter studies,[40,42,43] patients with positive, close or indetermi-

nate margins received more intensive radiotherapy (higher whole breast dosage and/or addition of a boost) than those with histologically negative margins. A more radical radiotherapeutic approach was apparently considered necessary to keep the risk of recurrence within acceptable limits. Pezner et al[38] reported an actuarial 48-month, 100% local control rate in 53 patients in whom the surgical margins were histopathologically tumor-free, and who received whole breast irradiation without a boost. This compares to 87% local control (p < 0.03) in 28 patients with unknown margin status who were treated with whole breast radiotherapy followed by an interstitial or electron beam boost.

Interestingly, series in which the microscopic status of surgical margins was not well documented[24,43,45-52] or which included patients with microscopically negative, indeterminate and positive margins[33,39] report that the presence of extensive intraductal carcinoma in association with the primary tumor (the so-called "extensive intraductal component" [EIC]) implies a significantly increased risk of ipsilateral breast tumor relapse after conservative treatment. This histological feature has been found to correlate with the presence of breast cancer multicentricity.[45,53,54] EIC is defined as ductal carcinoma in situ comprising at least 25% of the primary tumor area on histological sections and intraductal carcinoma extending beyond the infiltrating margin of the tumor or present in sections of grossly normal adjacent breast parenchyma.[55]

Careful analysis of the NSABP B-06 data failed to demonstrate any influence of EIC on risk for local recurrence.[56] This may well be because all patients in the breast conservation arms in this trial were required to have microscopically tumor-free lumpectomy margins.[43,57] In essence, when the histological status of surgical margins is either unknown or not specified as a criterion for adequacy of surgery, EIC may serve as a surrogate for microscopic margin involvement, and therefore as a measure of risk for residual tumor in the ipsilateral breast postoperatively.[58]

MULTICENTRICITY AND BREAST-CONSERVING SURGERY

The multifocal or multicentric nature of early breast cancer has long been cited by opponents of breast-conserving therapy as a rationale for avoidance of this option. The reported incidence in the literature of microscopic deposits of tumor cells some distance away from the main tumor mass varies greatly. Significant determinants of the incidence of multicentricity include the method used to measure it, the thoroughness with which it is sought, whether discontinuous foci of atypical hyperplasia are counted along with foci of in situ or invasive neoplasia, and inclusion of lobular carcinoma in situ (LCIS) lesions as multicentric foci of true neoplasia.[59] Atypical hyperplasias and LCIS are best regarded as markers of breast cancer risk; neither is clearly a precursor lesion in the classical sense (see chapter 8).

Analysis of the results of the NSABP B-04 trial, in which only a single randomly selected tissue block from one breast quadrant was examined per patient, revealed microscopic foci of multicentric cancer in 121 of 904 breasts (13.4%).[53] Statistically significant associations were found between multicentricity and tumor size greater than 5 cm, the presence of intraductal disease within and around the invasive tumor, tumor involvement of the nipple, and the presence of tumor emboli within the breast lymphatics.

In a histological study of serial whole-breast sections, Egan[60] reported multicentricity in 72 of 118 unilateral carcinomas (60%). In contrast, Lagios[54] using similar techniques found multicentricity in only 18 of 85 cases (21%); half of the separate foci were invasive carcinoma, and affected patients were more likely to have a family history of breast cancer or a contralateral breast cancer. Tubular carcinomas demonstrated a predilection for multicentricity.

In a study of simulated partial mastectomy (complete excision of all gross tumor with a margin of normal appearing breast tissue) in 203 total mastectomy specimens from breast cancer patients, Rosen et al[61] found residual infiltrating or in situ carcinoma in the remaining breast tissue in 26% of 100 specimens with tumors of less than 2 cm, and 38% of 103 specimens with larger cancers. The incidence of residual invasive disease was 11% for tumors of less than 0.9 cm in greatest dimension, 15% for lesions of 1 to 2 cm, 25% for tumors of 2.1 to 4.0 cm, and 43% for cancers of over 4.0 cm. Breasts from patients with subareolar lesions or a family history of breast cancer had a higher incidence of multicentricity.

In a more recent study in which the distribution of discontinuous foci of tumor was carefully mapped with respect to the primary tumor mass, Holland et al[62] demonstrated that such foci tend to cluster around the primary tumor in a manner more consistent with multifocality (within the vicinity of or same quadrant as the reference tumor) than multicentricity (diffuse involvement of the affected breast). Of the 282 invasive cancers studied by the Egan method, no separate tumor foci were found in 37%, tumor foci were present within 2 cm of the primary cancer in 20% and extended beyond 2 cm in the remaining 43%. Primary tumor size had no effect on the incidence of multifocality or distance of tumor foci from the reference cancer. Gump et al[59,63] in a subsequent systematic study of 657 breasts removed for palpable breast cancer also observed that 90% of discontinuous tumor foci were situated around the reference cancer in the 179 breasts (27%) in which multifocality was found. Significant correlations were found between multifocality and lobular or intraductal histology, and tumor size of over 2 cm.

The multicentric nature of breast cancer is disquieting in the context of breast-conserving therapy. In response to this concern, Fisher et al[56,64] looked for an association between ipsilateral breast tumor recurrence and multicentricity in the NSABP B-06 trial. At a mean followup of 103 months, recurrences had almost always occurred in close proximity to or within the same quadrant as the original primary cancer, and were of the same histological subtype and nuclear grade. The authors concluded that multicentricity has very limited clinical relevance, and the observations from the prospective trials reviewed in chapter 1 sustain this assessment. In these and most retrospective studies as well, the incidence of ipsilateral breast tumor recurrence following conservative treatment has been much lower than the reported frequency of multicentricity. Local recurrences are most often seen near or within the site of the original tumor, and tend to develop within the first five years of followup.[22,47,65,66]

There is a small but protracted risk (about 1% per annum) of recurrent ipsilateral breast cancer in locations remote from the original primary lesion;[47,65] these "treatment failures" are not infrequently of different grade and histological subtype as compared to the original cancer. They are somewhat analogous to metachronous contralateral breast cancer (see chapter 10) in that they probably represent new primaries and are clinical manifestations of multicentricity.[67]

A consensus has evolved among surgeons and radiotherapists that the use of breast-conserving treatment in patients with clinical, mammographic or gross pathological evidence of multifocal or multicentric breast cancer is ill-advised. There is therefore a paucity of experience from which to obtain information on the risk of local recurrence following conservative treatment of macroscopically multiple or synchronous ipsilateral breast cancers. Currently available data are summarized in Table 2.1.

In all three series, patients with two or more gross foci of disease had a substantially higher incidence of tumor relapse in the breast than those with unifocal tumors. Kurtz et al[45] noted that adequate margins (i.e. complete excision of all gross disease) were obtained in a significantly smaller proportion of patients with multifocal cancer. The effect of the gross status of the margins on local recurrence was highly significant by both univariate and multivariate analysis. Local failure occurred in 8 of 22 patients (36%) in whom multifocality was evident on clinical or mammographic examination, as compared to 7 of 39 patients (18%) in whom the multifocal nature of their disease was appreciated only on gross pathological examination. Only one of 21 bifocal tumors diagnosed by the pathologist recurred as compared to 6 of 18 tumors comprised of three or more separate nodules (p < 0.025). Of the 15 ipsilateral breast tumor recurrences in the 61 multifocal cancers in this series, only four occurred in the vicinity of the original disease. The other 11 recurrences were situated at a distance from the index lesions, or were diffuse or multifocal themselves. This was in contrast to the recurrences in the unifocal group, most of which were in or near the site of the original cancer.

It is apparent that patients with grossly multifocal breast cancer are indeed at substantially higher risk for local failure, and that the pattern of local recurrence differs

Table 2.1. Results of breast-conserving treatment in patients with macroscopically multicentric breast cancer

| | **Unifocal Cancers** | | **Multifocal Cancers** | | |
Series	No. Patients	No. IBTR*	No. Patients	No. IBTR*	Significance
Kurtz[45]	525	56 (11%)	61	15 (25%)	p < 0.005
Wilson[68]	1047	12%†	13	25%†	—
Leopod[69]	707	77 (11%)	10	4 (40%)	p = 0.019

* Ipsilateral breast tumor recurrence.
† These are 72-month actuarial local recurrence rates.

from that of unifocal disease. However, these limited data suggest that this risk is not absolutely prohibitive. Provided the tumor can be completely excised, it is not entirely unreasonable to attempt conservative surgical resection in selected, carefully counselled patients who have a strong aversion to total mastectomy.

RE-EXCISION OF THE BREAST TUMOR SITE AFTER BIOPSY OR TUMORECTOMY

Patients with excisional biopsy-proven invasive breast cancer require axillary lymphadenectomy for purposes of staging, adjuvant systemic therapy considerations and regional disease control. There often arises the question of whether further excision of breast tissue around the site of the primary tumor should be performed under the same anaesthetic.

The multicentricity data reviewed above suggest a definite potential for persistent residual disease when conservative surgery is performed for breast cancer. The study of simulated partial mastectomy by Rosen et al[61] demonstrated this particularly well. Frazier et al[70] analyzed breast re-excision specimens in 87 breast cancer patients in whom the status of margins of the initial breast specimen was classified microscopically by NSABP criteria. In 75 patients, the re-excision consisted of total mastectomy. Five of 19 patients (26%) with microscopically clear margins in the initial excision had further disease in the re-excision specimen. This figure approximates the 5-year incidence of local recurrence in patients in the B-06 trial treated by segmental mastectomy without radiation (Table 1.4). The re-excision specimens of nine of 28 patients (32.1%) in whom the initial margins were close and 21 of 40 patients (52%) with involved margins contained residual carcinoma. Eleven of the 75 mastectomy specimens had tumor in quadrants other than the one which harbored the original cancer.

In the series reported by McCormick et al,[32] of 33 patients whose initial conservative tumor excision was performed at an outside institution, re-excision yielded histopathological tumor-free margins in all but five.

Residual tumor was present in the re-excised breast tissue in 18 patients (invasive in 10 and noninvasive in 8).

Schnitt et al[52] and Solin et al[71] reported residual cancer in breast re-excisions in over 60% of patients in whom the second procedure was performed because of the presence of EIC or microscopically close or involved margins. Patients with EIC-positive lesions were especially likely to have residual tumor,[52] an observation in agreement with that of Holland et al.[58] Three of nine patients (33%) in whom the initial margins were clear had residual disease on re-excision. Morimoto et al[72] reported residual tumor over 2.6 cm from the site of the initial resection in re-excised breast specimens from 59 of 183 patients (32%).

Montague[73] examined the effect of re-excision on ipsilateral breast tumor recurrence rate. Among 135 patients in whom re-excision of the tumor site was not performed after referral to her institution, the recurrence rate was 8.2% as compared to a 2% incidence of breast relapse in 210 patients who underwent re-excision of the primary tumor site.

Taken together, these data suggest that re-excision of the site of the original primary cancer should at least be considered in candidates for breast-conserving therapy. If the biopsy has been performed by another surgeon, or if there is any question about the adequacy of tumor excision at the original procedure, most surgeons will re-excise the area en bloc with an ellipse of skin incorporating the biopsy scar.

RADIOTHERAPEUTIC CONSIDERATIONS

The proven value of postoperative adjuvant radiotherapy in reducing the risk of ipsilateral breast tumor relapse was addressed in the previous chapter (Table 1.4). There are a number of radiotherapy protocols which are commonly used at the present time, the differences between them relating to the type of breast-preserving operation performed, the status of the surgical margins, tumor size, whether adjuvant chemotherapy is to be administered, and other factors.

The physical and methodological advances in radiation oncology have greatly enhanced the effectiveness and utility of this therapeutic modality. Radiation-related acute toxicity in normal tissues is distinctly uncommon, and usually mild and transient when it does develop. Careful attention to treatment planning with exclusion of normal tissues from irradiation ports has reduced the occurrence of radiation pneumonitis and esophagitis to a minimum.[74]

WHOLE BREAST IRRADIATION

Adjuvant radiation therapy is usually started two to five weeks postoperatively. The whole breast is irradiated through medial and lateral tangential fields with the patient supine and the ipsilateral arm abducted over her head and held in an immobilization cast (Fig. 2.2). The tangential field irradiation is carried out using 4 to 8 MeV photons or Cobalt-60, and is given in 1.8 to 2.0 Gy fractions over 4 1/2 to 5 weeks to a total dose of 45 to 50 Gy.[74-78] This dosage range has been found to provide the optimal balance between tumor control and cosmetic outcome when the surgical procedure has been performed appropriately. Higher doses, especially in excess of 60 Gy, result in significant to severe sequelae in normal tissues which compromise the cosmetic result.[79] In obese patients or when the breast is large and/or fat-replaced, high energy photons (6 to 10 MeV) may provide better isodose distribution, resulting in less skin reaction and better cosmesis.[74,76]

Radiation exposure of the heart and lungs can be minimized by the use of half-beam blocks to eliminate posteriorly diverging radiation (Fig. 2.3), or by anterior angulation

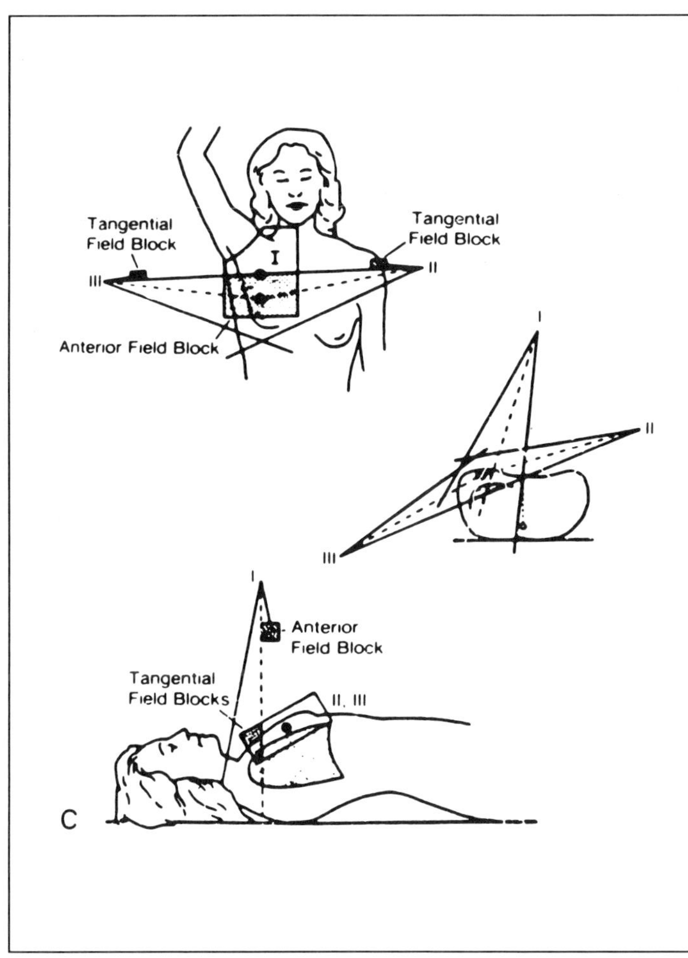

Fig. 2.2. Schematic depiction of the radiotherapy set-up for whole breast irradiation with an anterior field for supraclavicular nodal irradiation. Blocks are inserted in the superior margin of the tangential fields (II and III) and the inferior half of the supraclavicular field (I). The tangential beams are angled slightly caudad so that the upper edges of the beams are coincident. Similarly, angulation of the tangential beams anteriorly makes their posterior edges coincident, thereby minimizing irradiation of the lung and mediastinal structures. Reproduced with permission from Marcial VA. Cancer 1990; 65:2159-2164.

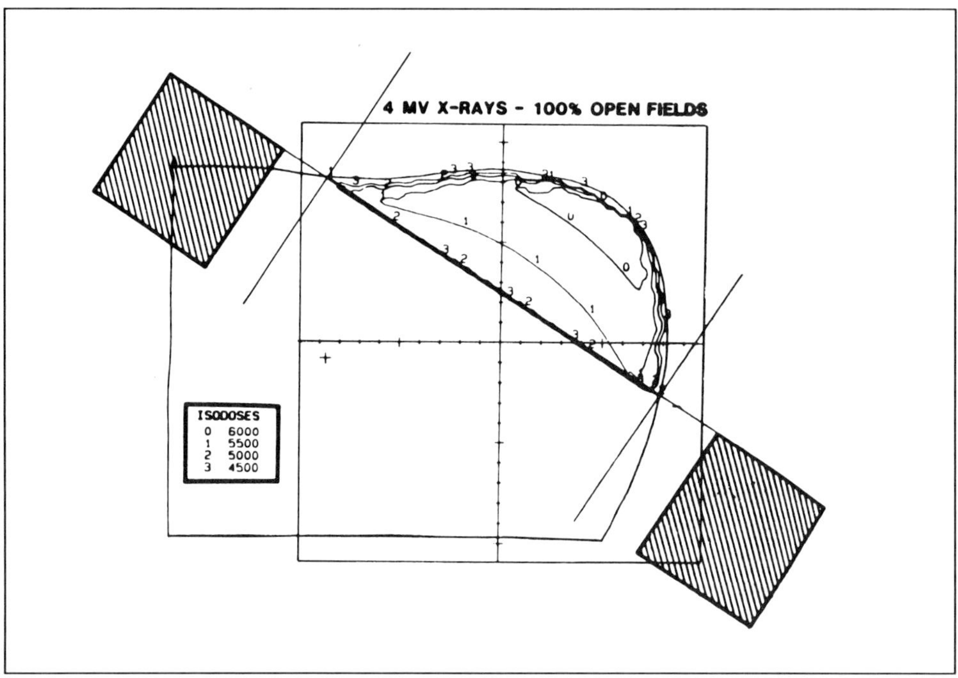

Fig. 2.3. A coronal view through the breast with the central axis of the tangential radiation fields shown. The half beam blocks (hatched squares) eliminate the posteriorly diverging radiation, thereby protecting the intrathoracic structures. Wedges are used anteriorly to improve the dose homogeneity in the breast tissue; without them, the anterior breast would receive excess irradiation, putting the patient at risk for a suboptimal cosmetic outcome. Reproduced with permission from Marcial VA. Cancer 1990; 65:2159-2164.

of the incident radiation beam. A minimum of 1.5 cm but no more than 3.5 cm of the underlying lung is included in the radiation field.[74]

The use of wedges in the anterior half of the beam may improve dose homogeneity, and thereby avoid excessive irradiation of the anterior portion of the breast.[77]

The weekly radiotherapy dose should be no less than 8 Gy to avoid a 25% or higher incidence of ipsilateral breast tumor recurrence.[80,81] If commencement of radiotherapy is delayed beyond the seventh postoperative week, local recurrence rates are also adversely affected.[41,82] Long term cosmesis may suffer if radiation fractions of 2.5 Gy or higher are used, or if the dosage to the whole breast exceeds 50 Gy by a significant amount.[75,77]

The radiotherapy protocol used in the NSABP B-06 trial consisted of only whole breast irradiation to 50 Gy in 25 fractions of 2 Gy each; irradiation of the regional lym-

phatics was avoided, and the tumor bed was not treated with a boost. Adoption of this regimen by the NSABP was based on the results of the B-04 trial, in which irradiation of the chest wall significantly reduced the incidence of local recurrence in both clinical node-negative and node-positive patients. Because histopathologically tumor-free margins were required in the B-06 trial, this regimen was deemed satisfactory for control of the primary tumor, and the results at 5, 8 and 9 years followup confirmed the validity of this assessment. The NSABP presently permits the use of a boost to the tumor bed, preferably with an external electron beam in 2 Gy fractions to a total additional dose of 10 to 20 Gy.[78]

RADIATION BOOST TO THE PRIMARY TUMOR SITE

The use of boosts when the surgical margins are histopathologically clear is of as yet unproven benefit.[74] The numbers of patients which would be necessary in a prospective clinical trial to demonstrate an advantage in these circumstances would likely have to be very large.[78]

However, boosting the radiation dosage to the tumor bed either by external beam or interstitial therapy in patients with microscopically close or involved margins significantly improves tumor control in the ipsilateral breast.[74-77,83] Failure to use a boost when the margins were histologically positive eventuated in a four-fold increase in incidence of local recurrence, in the experience of Ryoo et al.[75] So too, a boost may be indicated for patients with larger, macroscopically multiple or EIC-positive tumors.[45,84]

The boost dose can be administered either by external beam electrons or photons, or by brachytherapy. Each of these two approaches has advantages and weaknesses, and there are no data which clearly identify one as superior to the other either in terms of local recurrence or cosmetic outcome. External beam boosts are given with Cobalt-60, orthovoltage or low energy megavoltage equipment. The volume of the boost is carefully limited for cosmetic reasons. For small or well circumscribed cancers, 2 cm margins are planned while EIC-positive tumors may require a 3 cm margin. The boost dose is calculated from the deepest part of the tumor bed, and when electrons are used the energy chosen is that which encompasses this point with the 80% to 85% isodose line.[77]

The use of interstitial ^{192}Ir requires a general anaesthetic for insertion of after-loading catheters. This disadvantage is offset by the convenience of having the treatment completed over a very short period of time.

Irradiation of the Regional Lymphatics

Many centers irradiate one or more of the regional lymph node areas along with the breast. This practice is controversial, as prospective randomized trials such as NSABP B-04[85] and the Cancer Research Campaign trial[86] have demonstrated no survival benefit in patients so treated. As noted by Deutsch,[78] the incidence of first relapse in the supra-

clavicular region in clinical axillary node-positive patients randomized to radical mastectomy in the B-04 study was only 5.8%. It is noteworthy that the patients in this study received no adjuvant systemic therapy. Seven subsequent NSABP trials of various adjuvant chemotherapy regimens confirmed that the incidence of supraclavicular or internal mammary relapse is low.

It should be noted that these trials included only patients with pathological node-positive breast cancer, 50% of whom had more than four involved axillary nodes. Medial and central tumors were well represented (32% to 40% of patients in each trial) and followup has ranged from 6 to 16 years.

Furthermore, like chest wall recurrence following total mastectomy, supraclavicular and internal mammary nodal metastases are now recognized as manifestations of systemic dissemination, and affected patients are considered to have Stage IV disease. The management of such patients is palliative, and includes the use of radiotherapy, chemotherapy and endocrine manipulation.

When regional nodal irradiation is to be used in the postoperative adjuvant setting, careful planning is required as there is significant potential for field overlap with resultant cosmetic problems due to matchline fibrosis (Fig. 2.2). Problems related to lymphedema of the ipsilateral breast and arm are much more frequent when both surgery and radiation are employed in the management of the axillary lymphatics (see chapter 5). In the past, irradiation of the internal mammary lymphatics through an anterior or en face portal has resulted in chemotherapy dose-limiting leukopenia. This has been attributed to the unavoidable exposure of the heart, great vessels and a long segment of the thoracic vertebral bone marrow, with irradiation of the circulating blood volume with each treatment. There is a low but measurable excess risk of coronary artery disease related to such radiation techniques (vide infra). If the internal mammary nodes are to be irradiated, it is probably safer to do so by extending the tangential breast fields medially to include them (Fig. 2.4).[77-82,84-87]

Fig. 2.4. Comparison of an anterior internal mammary field (A) with extension of the tangential fields to include the internal mammary lymphatics (B). In A, much of the mediastinum and thoracic vertebral marrow are unavoidably irradiated, and the patient is at risk for matchline fibrosis at the points where the anterior field and tangential beams come together. These disadvantages can be largely obviated by the approach shown in B. Reproduced with permission from Bedwinek J. Cancer 1984; 53:729-739.

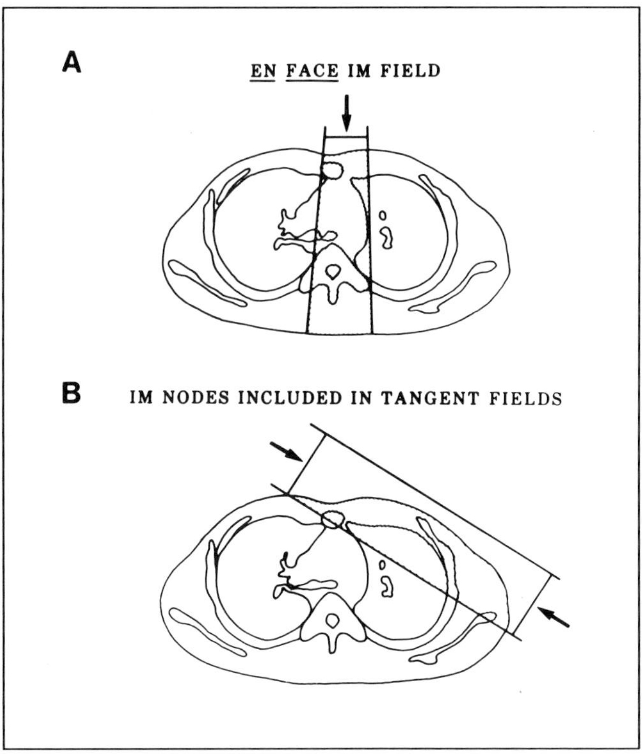

LONG TERM SEQUELAE OF BREAST-CONSERVING THERAPY

At the present time, the risk of serious long term consequences due to breast-conserving therapy appears to be very low. Concern has been expressed about the possibility of radiation-related carcinogenesis with new neoplasms arising within or near the treated tissue volume, or in the contralateral breast years to decades later. In addition, there is some evidence of a very small excess risk for coronary artery disease and other nonmalignant complications of normal tissue irradiation.

These complications have usually arisen many years to decades after treatment. The radiotherapy given for the original breast cancer was often orthovoltage or older megavoltage therapy, and administered with less precision, as regards normal tissue exclusion from radiation fields, than would now be done as a matter of routine. The literature on this subject must therefore be interpreted with considerable caution, as it has limited relevance to patients undergoing treatment today. With modern radio-therapeutic technology and advances in radiation planning, it is quite pos-sible that the rare occurrence of these complications as reported in the literature significantly overstates the risk for patients currently undergoing breast-conserving therapy.

LEUKEMOGENESIS

The NSABP reported a very small but statistically significant increase in excess risk for acute myelogenous leukemia among the 646 of 8,483 protocol patients in whom irradiation or chemotherapy was included as part of the treatment for their breast cancers.[88] In a study of 22,753 Connecticut Tumor Registry breast cancer cases diagnosed from 1935 to 1972, Curtis et al[89] attempted but were unable to confirm an association between radiotherapy and leukemia. In a subsequent case-control study in 82,700 breast cancer patients diagnosed between 1973 and 1985, they found that the relative risk of leukemia was 2.4 in patients treated with radiation, 10.0 in those who received chemotherapy, and 17.4 in patients treated with combined radiotherapy and chemotherapy. The mean estimated radiation dose to the bone marrow in studied patients was

7.5 Gy. Melphalan was by far the most leukemogenic agent studied; the risk of leukemia following standard cyclophosphamide regimens or radiotherapy was more modest, and the radiation effect correlated with cumulative bone marrow radiation dose.[90]

CONTRALATERAL BREAST CARCINOMA

Because of the well documented excess risk for breast cancer among atomic bomb survivors[91,92] and women irradiated for nonneoplastic medical conditions,[93-97] childhood cancer[98] or Hodgkin's disease,[99,100] there has been interest in evaluating whether adjuvant breast irradiation in breast cancer patients results in an excess risk for contralateral breast cancer. The excess risk of breast cancer was highest among women exposed to ionizing radiations at a young age.[94-100]

With current methods of irradiating the conserved breast, the opposite breast is unavoidably exposed to a low dose of ionizing radiations. The contralateral breast receives a minimum of 0.5 Gy[101] and may be exposed to 3% to 13%,[101-103] and occasionally to as much as 36%,[103] of the dose administered to the treated breast depending upon the radiation technique used.

The question of whether or not there is an excess risk for metachronous contralateral breast cancer associated with postoperative adjuvant radiation to the conserved breast is highly controversial. Numerous studies of relatively small numbers of patients have purported to demonstrate or eschew such an association. Affirmative studies[104,105] are open to challenge because of potential biases in the patients being studied. Negative studies[106-111] can generally be discounted on the basis of inadequate statistical power.

Three large population-based studies (27,000 to over 56,000 patients each) have found that adjuvant breast or chest wall radiotherapy for breast cancer augments the relative risk for a contralateral breast cancer by a modest increment.[112-114] That this difference can only be demonstrated in such large numbers of patients suggests that the magnitude of the carcinogenic effect is very small.

In a recent case-control study,[115] a small but significant increase in risk for metachronous contralateral breast cancer was demonstrated only among patients who were 45 years of age or younger at the time of treatment of their initial tumors by breast-conserving surgery and adjuvant radiotherapy. That this effect should be confined to younger patients is consistent with findings of other studies of radiation-related carcinogenesis.

SECOND CANCERS ARISING WITHIN THE TREATED TISSUE VOLUME

There continue to be reports of soft tissue sarcomas arising in irradiated tissues many years after axillary lymphadenectomy or irradiation for breast cancer.[79,116-124] The incidence of Stewart-Treves syndrome and postirradiation sarcoma is extremely low, but these lesions are noteworthy for their virulent clinical behavior and high risk for recurrence and metastasis despite aggressive treatment. Latency periods are long, and therefore younger breast cancer patients and those with a good prognosis are at risk.[124]

An increased incidence of squamous cell carcinoma, small cell carcinoma and adenocarcinoma of the ipsilateral lung was recently reported in patients treated with breast or chest wall radiation for breast cancer.[125] These data were taken from the Surveillance, Epidemiology and End Results Program of the National Cancer Institute for 1973 through 1986. The latency period for these tumors was 10 years. Radiation dose distribution analysis suggested that the ipsilateral lung in these patients received 33.6% of the prescribed whole breast dose for Cobalt-60 therapy and 21.5% when 6 MeV megavoltage therapy was used. The contralateral lung received 4.7% of the prescribed dose with Cobalt-60, and 1.2% with 6 MeV photons. As a number of these patients were treated with Cobalt-60 postmastectomy rather than after breast conservation, the authors noted that current radiation techniques probably result in much less irradiation of the ipsilateral lung.

CORONARY ARTERY DISEASE

An association between the use of postoperative adjuvant radiotherapy following mastectomy in breast cancer patients and late excess mortality due to cardiac disease has been documented in several long term studies.[105,111,126,127] The patients in these studies were treated mainly with orthovoltage radiotherapy, although a weaker association was still found in patients treated with Cobalt-60 and megavoltage photons.[105,111] Avoidance of high risk radiation fields (the anterior "hockey stick" for irradiation of ipsilateral internal mammary and supraclavicular nodal regions)[111,128,129] should mitigate the risk of accelerated coronary atherosclerosis and fatal myocardial infarction. It is not at all clear that the benefits of routine nodal irradiation outweigh the risks, including cardiac morbidity and mortality.[129]

Tangential whole breast fields often did not fully protect the heart in the past, especially when the left breast or chest wall was being treated.[105] Posterior half-beam blocks or anterior angulation of the tangential beams should minimize cardiac exposure to ionizing radiations.[77]

As the latency of the clinical manifestations of radiation on coronary atherosclerosis is long, younger patients and those with a good prognosis (and therefore a long life expectancy) are at risk. Once again, it must be stressed that much progress has been made in radiotherapy planning and treatment, and it is almost certain that a patient irradiated now has a far lower excess risk of myocardial infarction than a patient irradiated for breast cancer 20 years ago. The excess risk identified with these older techniques is itself very small.

Other Long term Sequelae

Late development of soft tissue necrosis in the chest wall, radiation-induced rib fractures, osteonecrosis and radiation-induced brachial plexopathies are infrequent occurrences in most series of breast cancer patients treated with adjuvant radiotherapy.[123,130-133] The risk of such complications is likely to continue to decrease as radiotherapy techniques undergo further refinement.

References

1. Atkins H, Hayward JL, Klugman DJ, Wayte AB. Treatment of early breast cancer: a report after ten years of a clinical trial. Br Med J 1972; 2:423-429.

2. Veronesi U, Saccozzi R, Del Vecchio M, et al. Comparing radical mastectomy with quadrantectomy, axillary dissection and radiotherapy in patients with small cancers of the breast. New Engl J Med 1981; 305: 6-11.

3. Uppsala-Örebro. Breast Cancer Study Group. Sector resection with or without postoperative radiotherapy for Stage I breast cancer: a randomized trial. J Natl Cancer Inst 1990; 82:277-282.

4. Crile G Jr. Simplified treatment of cancer of the breast: early results of a clinical study. Ann Surg 1975; 181:26-30.

5. Hermann RE, Esselstyn EB Jr., Cooperman AM, Crile G Jr. Partial mastectomy without radiation therapy. Surg Clin North Am 1984; 64:1103-1113.

6. Hermann RE, Esselstyn EB Jr., Grundfest-Broniatowski S, et al. Partial mastectomy without radiation is adequate treatment for patients with Stages 0 and I carcinoma of the breast. Surg Gynecol Obstet 1993; 177:247-253.

7. Hermann RE, Grundfest-Broniatowski S, Esselstyn CB Jr. Breast-conserving surgery: how much is enough? Semin Surg Oncol 1992; 8:136-139.

8. Fisher B, Bauer M, Margolese R, et al. Five-year results of a randomized clinical trial comparing total mastectomy and segmental mastectomy with or without radiation in the treatment of breast cancer. New Engl J Med 1985; 312:665-673.

9. Fisher B, Redmond C, Poisson R, et al. Eight-year results of a randomized trial comparing total mastectomy and lumpectomy with or without irradiation in the treatment of breast cancer. New Engl J Med 1989; 320:822-828.

10. Lichter AS, Lippman ME, Danforth DN Jr., et al. Mastectomy versus breast-conserving therapy in the treatment of Stage I and II carcinoma of the breast: a randomized trial of the National Cancer Institute. J Clin Oncol 1992; 10:976-983.

11. Straus K, Lichter A, Lippman M, et al. Results of the National Cancer Institute Early Breast Cancer Trial. J Natl Cancer Inst Monogr 1992; 11:27-32.

12. van Dongen JA, Bartelink H, Fentiman IS, et al. Randomized clinical trial to assess the value of breast-conserving therapy in Stage I and II breast cancer: EORTC 10801 trial. J Natl Cancer Inst Monogr 1992; 11:15-18.

13. Veronesi U, Volterrani F, Luini A, et al. Quadrantectomy versus lumpectomy for small size breast cancer. Eur J Cancer 1990; 26:671-673.

14. Ruffin WK, Wood WC. The role of surgery for early breast cancer. In: Ariel IM, Cahan AC, eds. Treatment of Precancerous Lesions and Early Breast Cancer. Baltimore: Williams & Wilkins, 1993:76-92.

15. Blichert-Toft M, Brincker H, Andersen JA, et al. A Danish randomized trial comparing breast-preserving therapy with mastectomy in mammary carcinoma. Acta Oncol 1988; 27:671-677.

16. Blichert-Toft M, Rose C, Andersen JA, et al. Danish randomized trial comparing breast conservation therapy with mastectomy: six years of life-table analysis. J Natl Cancer Inst Monogr 1992; 11:19-26.

17. Kurtz JM. Radiation therapy and breast preservation: past achievements, current results and future prospects. Semin Surg Oncol 1992; 8:147-152.

18. Leung S, Otmezguine Y, Calitchi E, et al. Locoregional recurrences following radical external beam irradiation and interstitial implantation for operable breast cancer - a twenty three year experience. Radiother Oncol 1986; 5:1-10.

19. Spitalier JM, Gambarelli J, Brandone H, et al. Breast-conserving surgery with radiation therapy for operable mammary carcinoma: a 25 year experience. World J Surg 1986; 10:1014-1020.

20. Pierquin B, Owen R, Maylin C, et al. Radical radiation therapy of breast cancer. Int J Radiat Oncol Biol Phys 1980; 6:17-24.

21. Amalric R, Santamaria F, Robert F, et al. Radiation therapy with or without primary limited surgery for operable breast cancer: a 20-year experience at the Marseilles Cancer Institute. Cancer 1982; 49:30-34.

22. Recht A, Silver B, Schnitt SJ, Connolly J, Hellman S, Harris JR. Breast relapse following primary radiation therapy for early breast cancer. I. Classification, frequency and salvage. Int J Radiat Oncol Biol Phys 1985; 11:1271-1276.

23. Calle R, Pilleron JP, Schlienger P, Vilcoq JR. Conservative management of operable breast cancer. Ten years experience at the Foundation Curie. Cancer 1978; 42: 2045-2053.

24. Schnitt SJ, Connolly J, Harris JR, Hellman S, Cohen RB. Pathologic predictors of early local recurrence in Stage I and II breast cancer treated by primary radiation therapy. Cancer 1984;53:1049-1057.

25. Van Limbergen E, Van der Schueren E, Van den Bogaert W, Van Wing J. Local control of operable breast cancer after radiotherapy alone. Eur J Cancer 1990; 26:674-679.

26. Vicini FA, Eberlein TJ, Connolly JL, et al. The optimal extent of resection for patients with Stages I or II breast cancer treated with conservative surgery and radiotherapy. Ann Surg 1991; 214:200-205.

27. Ghossein NA, Alpert S, Barba J, et al. Breast cancer. Importance of adequate surgical excision prior to radiotherapy in the local control of breast cancer in patients treated conservatively. Arch Surg 1992; 127: 411-415.

28. Gould EW, Robinson PG. The pathologist's examination of the "lumpectomy" -the pathologist's view of surgical margins. Semin Surg Oncol 1992; 8:129-135.

29. Rosen PP. Pathological assessment of non-palpable breast lesions. Semin Surg Oncol 1991; 7:257-260.

30. Carter D. Margins of "lumpectomy" for breast cancer. Hum Pathol 1986; 17: 330-332.

31. Fisher B, Wolmark N, Fisher ER, Deutsch M. Lumpectomy and axillary dissection for breast cancer: surgical, pathological, and radiation considerations. World J Surg 1985; 9:692-698.

32. McCormick B, Kinne D, Petrek J, et al. Limited resection for breast cancer: a study of inked specimen margins before radiotherapy. Int J Radiat Oncol Biol Phys 1987; 13:1667-1671.

33. Kurtz JM, Jacquemier J, Amalric R, et al. Why are local recurrences after breast-conserving therapy more frequent in younger patients? J Clin Oncol 1990; 8:591-598.

34. Anscher MS, Jones P, Prosnitz LR, et al. Local failure and margin status in early-stage breast carcinoma treated with conservation surgery and radiation therapy. Ann Surg 1993; 218:22-28.

35. Zafrani B, Vielh P, Fourquet A, et al. Conservative treatment of early breast cancer: prognostic value of ductal in situ component and other pathological variables on local control and survival. Eur J Cancer Clin Oncol 1989; 25:1645-1650.

36. Fourquet A, Campana F, Zafrani B, et al. Prognostic factors of breast recurrence in the conservative management of early breast cancer. Int J Radiat Oncol Biol Phys 1989; 17:719-725.

37. Hallahan DE, Michel AG, Halpern HJ, et al. Breast-conserving surgery and definitive irradiation for early breast cancer. Int J Radiat Oncol Biol Phys 1989; 17:1211-1216.

38. Pezner RD, Lipsett JA, Desai K, et al. To boost or not to boost: decreasing radiation therapy in conservative breast cancer treatment when "inked" tumor resection margins are pathologically free of cancer. Int J Radiat Oncol Biol Phys 1988; 14:873-877.

39. Kurtz JM, Jacquemier J, Amalric R, et al. Risk factors for breast recurrence in premenopausal and postmenopausal patients with ductal cancers treated by conservation therapy. Cancer 1990; 65:1867-1878.

40. Solin LJ, Fowble BL, Schultz DJ, Goodman RL. The significance of the pathology margins of the tumor excision on the outcome of patients treated with definitive irradiation of early breast cancer. Int J Radiat Oncol Biol Phys 1991; 21: 279-287.

41. Clarke DH, Le MG, Sarrazin D, et al. Analysis of local-regional relapses in patients with early breast cancers treated by excision and radiotherapy: experience of the Institut Gustave-Roussy. Int J Radiat Oncol Biol Phys 1985; 11:137-145.

42. Schmidt-Ullrich R, Wazer D, Tercilla O, et al. Tumor margin assessment as a guide to optimal conservation surgery and irradiation in early stage breast carcinoma. Int J Radiat Oncol Biol Phys 1989; 17: 733-738.

43. Bartelink H, Borger JH, van Dongen JA, Peterse JL. The impact of tumor size and histology on local control after breast-conserving therapy. Radiother Oncol 1988; 11:297-303.

44. Ryoo MC, Kagan AR, Wollin M, et al. Prognostic factors for recurrence and cosmesis in 393 patients after radiation therapy for early mammary carcinoma. Radiology 1989; 172:555-559.

45. Kurtz JM, Jacquemier J, Amalric R, et al. Breast-conserving therapy for macroscopically multiple cancers. Ann Surg 1990; 212:38-44.

46. Osteen RT, Connolly JL, Recht A, Silver B, Schnitt SJ, Harris JR. Identification of patients at high risk for local recurrence after conservative surgery and radiation therapy for stage I and II breast cancer. Arch Surg 1987; 122:1248-1252.

47. Recht A, Silen W, Schnitt SJ, et al. Time-course of local recurrence following conservative surgery and radiotherapy for early stage breast cancer. Int J Radiat Oncol Biol Phys 1988; 15:255-261.

48. Peterse JL, van Dongen JA, Bartelink H. Recurrence of breast carcinoma after breast-conserving therapy. Eur J Surg Oncol 1988; 14:123-126.

49. Harris JR, Connolly JL, Schnitt SJ, et al. The use of pathologic features in selecting the extent of surgical resection necessary for breast cancer patients treated by primary radiation therapy. Ann Surg 1985; 201: 164-169.

50. Recht A, Connolly JL, Schnitt SJ, et al. The effect of young age on tumor recurrence in the treated breast after conservative surgery and radiotherapy. Int J Radiat Oncol Biol Phys 1988; 14:3-10.

51. Harris JR, Connolly JL, Schnitt SJ, Cohen RB, Hellman S. Clinical -pathologic study of early breast cancer treated by primary radiation therapy. J Clin Oncol 1983; 1:184-189.

52. Schnitt SJ, Connolly JL, Khettry U, et al. Pathologic findings on re-excision of the primary site in breast cancer patients considered for treatment by primary radiation therapy. Cancer 1987; 59:675-681.

53. Fisher ER, Gregorio R, Redmond C, Vellios F, Sommers SC, Fisher B. Pathologic findings from the National Surgical Adjuvant Breast Project (Protocol No. 4). I. Observations concerning the multicentricity of mammary cancer. Cancer 1975; 35:247-254.

54. Lagios MD. Multicentricity of breast carcinoma demonstrated by routine correlated serial subgross and radiographic examination. Cancer 1977; 40:1726-1734.

55. Recht A, Connolly JL, Schnitt SJ, et al. Conservative surgery and radiation therapy for early breast cancer: results, controversies, and unsolved problems. Semin Oncol 1986; 13:434-449.

56. Fisher ER, Sass R, Fisher B, et al. Pathologic findings from the National Surgical Adjuvant Breast Project (Protocol No. 6). II. Relation of local recurrence to multicentricity. Cancer 1986; 57:1717-1724.

57. Margolese R. Surgical considerations in selecting local therapy. J Natl Cancer Inst Monogr 1992; 11:41-48.

58. Holland R, Connolly JL, Gelman R, et al. The presence of an extensive intraductal component following a limited excision correlates with prominent residual disease in the remainder of the breast. J Clin Oncol 1990; 8:113-118.

59. Gump FE. Multicentricity in early breast cancer. Semin Surg Oncol 1992; 8:117-121.

60. Egan RL. Multicentric breast carcinomas. Clinical-radiographic-pathologic whole organ studies and 10 year survival. Cancer 1982; 49:1123-1130.

61. Rosen PP, Fracchia AA, Urban JA, Schottenfeld D, Robbins GF. "Residual" mammary carcinoma following simulated partial mastectomy. Cancer 1975; 35:739-747.

62. Holland R, Veling SHJ, Mravunac M, Hendriks JHCL. Histologic multifocality of Tis, T1-2 breast carcinomas. Implications for clinical trials of breast-conserving surgery. Cancer 1985;56:979-990.

63. Gump FE, Habif DV, Logerfo P, et al. The extent and distribution of cancer in breasts with palpable primary tumors. Ann Surg 1986; 204:384-390.

64. Fisher ER, Anderson S, Redmond C, Fisher B. Ipsilateral breast tumor recurrence and survival following lumpectomy and irradiation: pathological findings from NSABP protocol B-06. Semin Surg Oncol 1992; 8:161-166.

65. Kurtz JM, Amalric R, Brandone H, et al. Local recurrence after breast-conserving surgery and radiotherapy. Cancer 1989; 63:1912-1917.

66. Harris JR, Recht A, Amalric R, et al. Time course and prognosis of local recurrence following primary radiation therapy for early breast cancer. J Clin Oncol 1984; 2:37-41.

67. Moffat FL, Ketcham AS, Robinson DS, et al. Segmental mastectomy without radiotherapy for T1 and small T2 breast carcinomas. Arch Surg 1990; 125:364-369.

68. Wilson LD, Beinfeld M, McKhann CF, Haffty BG. Conservative surgery and radiation in the treatment of synchronous ipsilateral breast cancers. Cancer 1993; 72:137-142.

69. Leopold KA, Recht A, Schnitt SJ, et al. Results of conservative surgery and radiation therapy for multiple synchronous cancers of one breast. Int J Radiat Oncol Biol Phys 1989; 16:11-16.

70. Frazier TG, Wong RWY, Rose D. Implications of accurate pathologic margins in the treatment of primary breast cancer. Arch Surg 1989; 124:37-38.

71. Solin LJ, Fowble B, Martz K, et al. Results of re-excisional biopsy of the primary tumor in preparation for definitive irradiation of patients with early stage breast cancer. Int J Radiat Oncol Biol Phys 1986; 12:721-725.

72. Morimoto T, Okazaki K, Komaki K, et al. Cancerous residue in breast-conserving surgery. J Surg Oncol 1993; 52:71-76.

73. Montague ED. Conservation surgery and radiation therapy in the treatment of operable breast cancer. Cancer 1984; 53:700-704.

74. Winchester PD, Cox JD. Standards for breast-conservation treatment. CA - A Cancer Journal for Clinicians 1992; 42:134-162.

75. Fowble B. Radiotherapeutic considerations in the treatment of primary breast cancer. J Natl Cancer Inst Monogr 1992; 11:49-58.

76. McCormick B. Radiation therapy in breast conservation patients and postmastectomy. Semin Surg Oncol 1991; 7:278-282.

77. Marcial VA. Primary therapy for limited breast cancer. Cancer 1990; 65:2159-2164.

78. Deutsch M. Radiotherapy after breast-conservation surgery: how much is enough? Semin Surg Oncol 1992; 8:140-146.

79. Delouche G, Bachelot F, Premont MD, Kurtz JM. Conservation treatment of early breast cancer: long term results and complications. Int J Radiat Oncol Biol Phys 1987; 13:29-34.

80. Kurtz JM, Spitalier J, Amalric R. Late breast recurrence after lumpectomy and irradiation. Int J Radiat Oncol Biol Phys 1983; 9: 1191-1194.

81. Osborne MP, Ormiston N, Harmer CL, et al. Breast conservation in the treatment of early breast cancer. Cancer 1984; 53:349-355.

82. Harter K, Goldberg R, Bryne P, et al. Local recurrence of breast cancer following lumpectomy in patients receiving adjuvant chemotherapy prior to definitive breast irradiation. Proc Amer Soc Clin Oncol 1984; 3:125 (Abstr).

83. Clark RM, Wilkinson RH, Miceli PN, MacDonald WD. Breast cancer: experiences with conservation therapy. Amer J Clin Oncol 1987; 10:461-468.

84. Dusenbery KE, Levitt SH. The role of conservative surgery and radiation therapy for early breast cancer. In: Ariel IM, Cahan AC, eds. Treatment of Precancerous Lesions and Early Breast Cancer. Baltimore: Williams and Wilkins, 1993:123-143.

85. Fisher B, Redmond C, Fisher ER, et al. Ten-year results of a randomized clinical trial comparing radical mastectomy and total mastectomy with or without radiation. New Engl J Med 1985; 312:674-681.

86. Baum M, Haybittle JL, Berstock DA, et al. Cancer Research Campaign trial for early breast cancer: a detailed update at the tenth year. Lancet 1980; 2:55-60.

87. Bedwinek J. Adjuvant irradiation for early breast cancer. An ongoing controversy. Cancer 1984; 53:729-739.

88. Fisher B, Rockette H, Fisher ER, et al. Leukemia in breast cancer patients following adjuvant chemotherapy or postoperative radiation: the NSABP experience. J Clin Oncol 1985; 3:1640-1658.

89. Curtis RE, Boice JD, Stovall M, Flannery JT, Moloney WC. Leukemia risk following radiotherapy for breast cancer. J Clin Oncol 1989; 7:21-29.

90. Curtis RE, Boice JD, Stovall M, et al. Risk of leukemia after chemotherapy and radiation treatment for breast cancer. New Engl J Med 1992; 326:1745-1751.

91. McGregor DH, Land CE, Choi K, et al. Breast cancer incidence among atomic bomb survivors, Hiroshima and Nagasaki, 1950-69. J Natl Cancer Inst 1977; 59:799-811.

92. Tokunaga M, Norman JE, Asano M, et al. Malignant breast tumors among atomic bomb survivors, Hiroshima and Nagasaki, 1950-74. J Natl Cancer Inst 1979; 62: 1347-1359.

93. Hoffman DA, Lonstein JE, Morin MM, et al. Breast cancer in women with scoliosis exposed to multiple diagnostic X-rays. J Natl Cancer Inst 1989; 81:1307-1312.

94. Baral E, Larsson L-E, Mattsson B. Breast cancer following irradiation of the breast. Cancer 1977; 40:2905-2910.

95. Shore RE, Hempelmann LH, Kowaluk E, et al. Breast neoplasms in women treated with X-rays for acute postpartum mastitis. J Natl Cancer Inst 1977; 59:813-822.

96. Boice JD, Monson RR. Breast cancer in women after repeated fluoroscopic examinations of the chest. J Natl Cancer Inst 1977; 59:823-832.

97. Land CE, Boice JD, Shore RE, Norman JE, Tokunaga M. Breast cancer risk from low-dose exposures to ionizing radiation: results of parallel analysis of three exposed populations of women. J Natl Cancer Inst 1980; 65:353-376.

98. Li FP, Corkery J, Vawter G, Fine W, Sallan SE. Breast carcinoma after cancer therapy in childhood. Cancer 1983; 51:521-523.

99. Yahalom J, Petrek JA, Biddinger PW, et al. Breast cancer in patients irradiated for Hodgkin's disease: a clinical and pathologic analysis of 45 events in 37 patients. J Clin Oncol 1992; 10:1674-1681.

100. Hancock SL, Tucker MA, Hoppe RT. Breast cancer after treatment of Hodgkin's disease. J Natl Cancer Inst 1993; 85:25-31.

101. Fraas BA, Roberson PL, Lichter AS. Dose to the contralateral breast die to primary breast irradiation. Int J Radiat Oncol Biol Phys 1985; 11:485-497.

102. Svensson GK, Kase KR, Chin LM, Harris JR. Dose to the opposite breast as a result of primary radiation therapy for carcinoma of the breast. Int J Radiat Oncol Biol Phys 1981; 7:1209 (Abstr).

103. Muller-Runkel R, Kalokhe UP. Scatter dose from tangential breast irradiation to the uninvolved breast. Radiology 1990; 175:873-876.

104. Brinkley D, Haybittle JL. A 15 year followup study of patients treated for carcinoma of the breast. Br J Radiol 1968; 41:215-221.

105. Haybittle JL, Brinkley D, Houghton J, A'Hern RP, Baum M. Postoperative radiotherapy and late mortality: evidence from the Cancer Research Campaign trial for early breast cancer. Br Med J 1989; 298: 1611-1614.

106. McCredie JA, Inch WR, Alderson M. Consecutive primary carcinomas of the breast. Cancer 1975; 35:1472-1477.

107. Basco VE, Coldman AJ, Elwood JM, Young MEJ. Radiation dose and second breast cancer. Br J Cancer 1985; 52:319-325.

108. Kurtz JM, Amalric R, Delouche G, et al. The second ten years: long-term risks of breast conservation in early breast cancer. Int J Radiat Oncol Biol Phys 1987; 13:1327-1332.

109. Kurtz JM, Amalric R, Brandone H, Ayme Y, Spitalier J-M. Contralateral breast cancer and other second malignancies in patients treated by breast-conserving therapy with radiation. Int J Radiat Oncol Biol Phys 1988; 15:277-284.

110. Lavey RS, Eby NL, Prosnitz LR. Impact of radiation therapy and/or chemotherapy on the risk for a second malignancy after breast cancer. Cancer 1990; 66:874-881.

111. Høst H, Brennhovd IO, Loeb M. Postoperative radiotherapy in breast cancer - long term results from the Oslo study. Int J Radiat Oncol Biol Phys 1986; 12:727-732.

112. Storm HH, Jensen OM. Risk of contralateral breast cancer in Denmark 1943-80. Br J Cancer 1986; 54:483-492.

113. Hankey BF, Curtis RE, Naughton MD, Boice JD, Flannery JT. A retrospective cohort analysis of second breast cancer risk for primary breast cancer patients with an assessment of the effect of radiation therapy. J Natl Cancer Inst 1983; 70:797-804.

114. Harvey EB, Brinton LA. Second cancer following cancer of the breast in Connecticut, 1935-1982. J Natl Cancer Inst Monogr 1985; 68:99-112.

115. Boice JD Jr., Harvey EB, Blettner M, Stovall M, Flannery JT. Cancer in the contralateral breast after radiotherapy for breast cancer. New Engl J Med 1992; 326:781-785.

116. Kuten A, Sapir D, Cohen Y, Borovik R, Robinson E. Postirradiation soft tissue sarcoma occurring in breast cancer patients: report of seven cases and results of combination chemotherapy. J Surg Oncol 1985; 28:168-171.

117. Hardy TJ, An T, Brown PW, Terz JJ. Postirradiation sarcoma (malignant fibrous histiocytoma) of axilla. Cancer 1978; 42:118-124.

118. Stokkel MPM, Peterse HL. Angiosarcoma of the breast after lumpectomy and radiation therapy for adenocarcinoma. Cancer 1992; 69:2965-2968.

119. Otis CN, Peschel R, McKhann C, Merino MJ, Duray PH. The rapid onset of cutaneous angiosarcoma after radiotherapy for breast carcinoma. Cancer 1986; 57: 2130-2134.

120. Ferguson DJ, Sutton HG, Dawson PJ. Late effects of adjuvant radiotherapy for breast cancer. Cancer 1984; 54:2319-2323.

121. Taghian A, de Vathaire F, Terrier P, et al. Long-term risk of sarcoma following radiation treatment for breast cancer. Int J Radiat Oncol Biol Phys 1991; 21:361-367.

122. Edeiken S, Russo DP, Knecht J, Parry LA, Thompson RM. Angiosarcoma after tylectomy and radiation therapy for carcinoma of the breast. Cancer 1992; 70:644-647.

123. Wang EHM, Sekyi-Otu A, O'Sullivan B, Bell RS. Management of long-term postirradiation periclavicular complications. J Surg Oncol 1992; 51:259-265.

124. Brady MS, Garfein CF, Petrek JA, Brennan MF. Posttreatment sarcoma in breast cancer patients. Ann Surg Oncol 1994; 1:66-72.

125. Neugut AI, Robinson E, Lee WC, et al. Lung cancer after radiation therapy for breast cancer. Cancer 1993; 71:3054-3071.

126. Cuzick J, Stewart H, Peto R, et al. Overview of randomized trials of postoperative adjuvant radiotherapy in breast cancer. Cancer Treat Rep 1987; 71:15-29.

127. Jones JM, Ribeiro GG. Mortality patterns over 34 years of breast cancer patients in a clinical trial of postoperative radiotherapy. Clin Radiol 1989; 40:204-208.

128. Harris JR, Hellman S. Put the "hockey stick" on ice. Int J Radiat Oncol Biol Phys 1988; 15:497-499.

129. Ebbs SR, Yarnold JR. Patient and anatomical selectivity in postoperative radiotherapy for early breast cancer: a British perspective. Semin Surg Oncol 1992; 8:167-171.

130. Kurtz JM, Amalric R, Delouche, et al. The second ten years: long-term risks of breast conservation in early breast cancer. Int J Radiat Oncol Biol Phys 1987; 13: 1327-1332.

131. Salner AL, Botnick LE, Herzog AG, et al. Reversible brachial plexopathy following primary radiation therapy for breast cancer. Cancer Treat Rep 1981; 65:797-801.

132. Match RM. Radiation-induced brachial plexus paralysis. Arch Surg 1975; 110: 384-386.

133. Bagley FH, Walsh JW, Cady B, Salzman FA, Oberfield RA, Pazianos AG. Carcinomatous versus radiation-induced brachial plexus neuropathy in breast cancer. Cancer 1978; 41:2154-2157.

CHAPTER 3

TUMOR RECURRENCE IN THE CONSERVED BREAST

Control of locoregional disease in patients with early breast cancer is critically important. Both radical surgery and breast-conserving therapy are attended by the infrequent but vexacious occurrence of locoregional tumor relapse.

Local failure often means loss of the affected breast, defeating the purpose of conservative breast cancer treatment. These occurrences may result in significant morbidity and can be profoundly detrimental to patients' peace of mind, quite apart from any effects on survival. For patients in whom the original carcinoma was managed by radical or modified radical mastectomy, locoregional relapse is usually the harbinger of eventual breast cancer mortality.

Substantial portions of the preceeding chapters were indirectly devoted to discussion of locoregional recurrence and breast-conserving therapy; local failure was considered from the standpoint of surgery, radiotherapy and adjuvant systemic therapy. In this chapter, the incidence, risk factors for and biological significance of tumor recurrence in the conserved breast or chest wall will be addressed. Salvage of ipsilateral breast tumor recurrence will also be discussed.

INCIDENCE OF IPSILATERAL BREAST TUMOR RECURRENCE

When breast conservation therapy was first used to treat early breast cancer, fear of an unacceptably high incidence of locoregional tumor recurrence was behind much of the opposition to this new treatment philosophy. It was held that the incidence of local failure would be prohibitive in the face of less than ablative surgery. As evidenced by findings of prospective and retrospective studies (Table 3.1), this contention proved to be without foundation. With appropriate conservative surgery and adjuvant radiotherapy, the risk of ipsilateral breast tumor recurrence is low; most patients who are considered candidates for and choose conservative treatment never experience breast cancer recurrence within the breast or the regional lymphatics.

The information given in Table 3.1 has been greatly simplified for the purpose of summarizing the reported incidence of local recurrence following breast-conserving therapy. The influence of various patient and tumor parameters, surgical particulars, type of radiation boost, regional nodal irradiation and adjuvant systemic therapy has largely been ignored. Nonetheless, this table not only reflects the tremendous diversity of breast conservation

Table 3.1. Incidence of local (ipsilateral breast) tumor recurrence in patients treated by breast conservation

Series	No. Patients	Surgery	Radiotherapy Whole Breast/Boost	Followup	Incidence of Local Recurrence
Gross Excision + Radiation					
EORTC 10801[1]	452	Tu	50 Gy/25 Gy	8 yrs	13%
DBCG-82TM[2]	430	Tu	50 Gy/10-25 Gy	40 mos	3%
U.S. NCI[3]	121	Tu	48.6 Gy/15-20 Gy	5 yrs	12%
				8 yrs	20%
Haffty[4]	278	Tu	46 Gy/10-20 Gy	5 yrs	9%
				10 yrs	20%
Calle[5]	324	Tu	50 Gy/10-15 Gy	5 yrs	8%
Chauvet[6]	202	Tu	45 Gy/15 Gy	5 yrs	14%
Kurtz[7]	1593	Tu	50-60 Gy/20-25 Gy	5 yrs	7%
				10 yrs	14%
				15 yrs	18%
				20 yrs	20%
Clark[8]	982	Tu	40 Gy/2.5-15 Gy	10 yrs	14%
Barr[9]	411	Tu	48.4 Gy/20 Gy	5 yrs	12%
				10 yrs	14%
Recht[10]	366	Tu	45-50 Gy/10-30 Gy	5 yrs	9%
Vicini[11]	1396	Tu	45-50 Gy/10-15 Gy	5 yrs	9%
				10 yrs	16%
Microscopically Clear Margins + Radiation					
NSABP B-06[12-16]	568	SM	50 Gy/None	5 yrs	8%
				8 yrs	11%
				9 yrs	12%
Hallahan[17]	219	SM	46 Gy/14-18 Gy	5 yrs	8%
Surgery Only, No Radiation*					
NSABP B-06[12-16]	572	SM	—	5 yrs	28%
				8 yrs	39%
				9 yrs	43%
Nemoto[18]	122	SM	—	4 yrs	18%
Lagios[19]	43	SM	—	2 yrs	19%
Clark[20]	374	Tu	—	5 yrs	25%
				10 yrs	28%
Montgomery[21]	31	Tu	—	3 yrs	28%

Tu   tumorectomy (clearance of gross disease only)
SM   segmental mastectomy (microscopic tumor-free margins)
* in unselected patients (i.e. without regard for risk factors for local recurrence)

protocols in use worldwide but also highlights the fact that, when appropriate combinations of conservative surgery and adjuvant radiotherapy are employed, the likelihood of local failure is both low and remarkably constant despite therapeutic variations among series.

A number of series report information on local recurrence in patients undergoing conservative surgery without breast irradiation. Prospective randomized data pertinent to this question were summarized in Table 1.5, and additional retrospective information is given in Table 3.1. When selected by the same criteria as those used for breast-conserving surgery plus adjuvant radiotherapy, patients treated by conservative surgery without breast irradiation have a much higher incidence of ipsilateral breast tumor recurrence, although the recurrence rate at ten years is still less than 50%. Adjuvant radiotherapy is very important for optimal locoregional disease control in breast conservation. The efficacy of this modality makes conservative management a viable alternative for a much larger proportion of breast cancer patients than might otherwise be appropriate.

DETECTION OF IPSILATERAL BREAST TUMOR RECURRENCE

Detection of recurrent cancer in the ipsilateral breast can be difficult in some patients.[21] Fortunately, treatment-related changes in the conserved breast are usually only minor to moderate in degree. The problems presented by these changes in the course of surveillance are manageable most of the time.

A few patients, mainly those with fair or poor cosmetic outcomes, present clinicians and radiologists with a formidable surveillance challenge. In these individuals, combined surgery and radiation results in moderate to marked dermal and parenchymal edema (early) and fibrosis (late) throughout the treated breast.[22-29] These changes are often most striking in the immediate vicinity of the surgical excision, the portion of the breast most at risk for tumor recurrence. Radiation dose inhomogeneities, especially in large or fat-replaced breasts, can result in fat necrosis which is clinically and mammographically indistinguishable from carcinoma.[26-29] These phenomena may compromise or even confound the clinician's and radiologist's ability to detect recurrent or new primary neoplasms in the affected breast.

The adverse influence of breast cancer surgery and radiotherapy on detection of tumor relapse is reflected in a significant impairment of the accuracy of mammographic surveillance following breast-conserving therapy. Mammography by itself may fail to detect 25% to over 50% of ipsilateral breast tumor recurrences because of treatment-induced changes in the radiographic appearance of the treated breast.[32-34] However, ipsilateral breast tumor recurrence is still detected solely by mammographic followup in approximately 20% to 40% of cases.

Recurrent tumor is often recognized radiographically by interval development of microcalcifications without, or less commonly with, an associated soft tissue density.[4,35-37] Mammographically-detected recurrences frequently presented as soft tissue mass lesions without microcalcification in one series.[38] Most recurrences detected only by mammography consisted predominantly or entirely of in situ cancer, in two series.[37,38] Fowble et al[36] noted that recurrence within the first five years after breast-conserving therapy was detected more often by mammography alone (41%) than late breast failures (8%).

All other recurrences present as palpable masses or nondescript thickenings in the breast. In one- to two-thirds of these cases, suspicious mammographic changes are also present. Thus, as in the initial detection of breast cancer, both mammographic surveillance and followup by serial physical examination are very important for timely diagnosis of disease recurrence in the ipsilateral breast.

Increased cicatricial reaction and fat necrosis sometimes eventuate in clinical and mammographic changes which cannot be ignored or simply observed, given the patient's history of ipsilateral breast cancer. Needle aspiration cytology may be difficult to interpret in the setting of previous irradiation and surgery, and in any event an inconclusive or negative cytological interpretation often mandates histological corroboration, particularly if the abnormality persists. In this small minority of affected patients, the surgeon is forced to resort to open biopsy more often than he or she otherwise might.[27,29]

Such biopsies may be complicated by wound healing problems and are detrimental to cosmesis. Because of the exaggerated fibrotic response seen in these wounds, the ability to detect interval development of tumor recurrence is further hindered. Pezner et al[30] reported the results of 27 open biopsies of the ipsilateral breast and axilla for benign abnormalities in 25 of 237 patients who had previously undergone conservative treatment for Stage I and II cancer. On histopathology, cutaneous or parenchymal fibrosis was found in eight, fat necrosis in seven and suture granulomas in three. Wound infection complicated eight of the 27 biopsies; of these, three healed within a month, four required three to seven months for omplete healing and the remaining patient developed a chronic, nonhealing ulcer. Significant correlates of wound healing complications included large breast size and removal of skin sutures less than 10 days postoperatively. Patients who underwent needle localization biopsy and those who had incisional skin biopsies for fibrotic changes had the highest incidence of complications (three of five and two of five, respectively). Three of the 17 (18%) excisional biopsies performed for palpable masses, and for which needle localization was therefore not required, developed complications. Solin et al[31] reported complications in 20% of needle localization biopsies and 8% of excisional biopsies in their series.

Cosmetic deterioration after biopsy of the conserved breast was seen in two of the eight patients in whom wound healing complications developed after open biopsy. In two others, mild retraction and telangiectasia developed at the biopsy site, and one was left with a nonhealing ulcer as already noted. Of the 17 patients whose open biopsies healed without complication, significant retraction developed in one and telangiectasia in one.[30]

Thus, a small number of patients pose very significant challenges to clinicians and radiologists related to surveillance for ipsilateral breast tumor recurrence. On rare occasions, intractable wound complications, biopsy-induced cosmetic deterioration and inability to evaluate such a breast have necessitated completion total mastectomy in the absence of recurrent cancer.[27]

RISK FACTORS FOR IPSILATERAL BREAST TUMOR RECURRENCE FOLLOWING BREAST-CONSERVING THERAPY

There has been much interest in the recent literature in identifying patient and tumor characteristics which influence the risk of local recurrence in the setting of breast-conserving therapy. Variables which have thus far been implicated as risk factors are discussed below.

The effects of treatment on ipsilateral breast tumor recurrence have already been reviewed in depth in chapter 2, and have also been reviewed by Kurtz.[39] The following discussion focuses on clinical, pathological and biochemical factors which may influence the risk of tumor recurrence in the ipsilateral breast.

AGE AND MENOPAUSAL STATUS

Patients of less than 35 to 40 years of age have been identified as being at higher risk for relapse of tumor in the breast in several series.[5,8,18,40-46] Clarke et al[47] found no association between age and ipsilateral breast recurrence. Several more recent studies have suggested that most of the excess risk ascribed to young age may in fact be attributable to a preponderance of extensive intraductal component, peritumor mononuclear cell reaction or high tumor grade in young breast cancer patients.[48-53] Age per se may or may not be a significant independent risk factor for local recurrence after breast-conserving therapy.

Premenopausal status has similarly been implicated,[5,42,54] but as with young age there may be other influences at work.[47]

SURGICAL MARGINS

The status of the surgical margins was discussed in detail in the previous chapter. It is abundantly clear that at a minimum, excision of all gross disease in the breast is essential for optimal control of the primary tumor. The presence of gross tumor involving one or more surgical margins around the primary cancer implies a four- to five-fold increase in risk of recurrence due to residual tumor even in the face of adequate radiation therapy to the breast.

There is no clear consensus regarding the importance of the microscopic status of the surgical margins, although most oncologists would agree that histopathological tumor-free margins are certainly desirable. Traditional principles of cancer surgery would hold that whenever possible, complete tumor excision as evidenced by microscopically negative resection margins should be sought for optimal local tumor control. A number of studies suggest that a histologically complete tumor excision yields a tangible benefit in terms of control of tumor in the breast (chapter 2).

PRIMARY TUMOR MULTICENTRICITY

This has also been discussed in the previous chapter. Gross multicentricity, while not an absolute contraindication to breast-conserving therapy, connotes an increased risk for local recurrence (Table 2.1). Paterson et al[55] reported that microscopic and gross multicentric disease was associated with a higher incidence of breast failure in their series.

PRIMARY TUMOR SIZE

Primary tumor size influences long term survival,[56] and affects both the extent of excision and the likelihood of complete removal of the primary cancer in a breast-conserving operation. As tumor size increases, so does the incidence of multicentricity.[57] In the National Surgical Adjuvant Breast Project (NSABP) B-06 trial, primary tumors of 2-cm diameter or larger had a significantly higher incidence of local relapse than smaller lesions in patients treated by segmental mastectomy without radiotherapy, but not in patients randomized to the segmental mastectomy plus radiotherapy arm.[58,59] Tumor size of over 2 cm was also a significant risk factor for local failure in the European Organization for Research and Treatment of Cancer (EORTC) 10801 trial,[1] in which all patients in the breast conservation arm underwent both surgical excision and adjuvant radiotherapy. Risk of local recurrence has also been found to correlate with tumor size in a number of retrospective analyses.[15,18,40,49,50,60]

EXTENSIVE INTRADUCTAL COMPONENT

This factor was briefly addressed in chapter 2. Extensive intraductal component (EIC) has been defined as "intraductal carcinoma comprising 25% or more of the (histological) area of the primary tumor mass and clearly extending beyond the infiltrating margin of the tumor or present in sections of grossly normal adjacent breast tissue"[61] (Fig. 3.1). The presence of EIC is indicative of a high probability of significant multicentricity[57,62,63] and implies an increased risk of ipsilateral breast tumor relapse in patients undergoing conservative treatment.[11,19,41-44,46,48,50,51,62,64-72] In addition, EIC has been identified as part of two constellations of variables (EIC plus high nuclear grade[67] and EIC plus peritumor mononuclear cell reaction in premenopausal patients[50]) which are associated with a very high risk of local recurrence.

However, EIC has only been identified as a significant risk factor for breast relapse in studies in which only gross tumor excision was required. EIC was not a significant factor in local recurrences in the NSABP B-06 trial, in which histopathological tumor-free margins were stipulated.[58] EIC may be a surrogate measure of adequacy of excision when the microscopic status of the surgical margins is not evaluated; when the margins are histopathologically clear of tumor, the presence or absence of EIC may have little or no bearing on the risk for local failure.

TUMOR GRADE

High grade or poorly differentiated tumors, as defined by Bloom and Richardson,[43,73] have a poorer prognosis than intermediate or low grade lesions. A number of recent reports have implicated high tumor grade as a risk factor for ipsilateral breast tumor recurrence following conservative treatment of early breast cancer.[15,47,48,50,54,58,59,67,69,74,75] Tumor necrosis, one of the criteria for high tumor grade, has also been cited as a risk factor for local failure,[50,76] although the NSABP[58] and Kurtz et al[48] found no evidence for such an association.

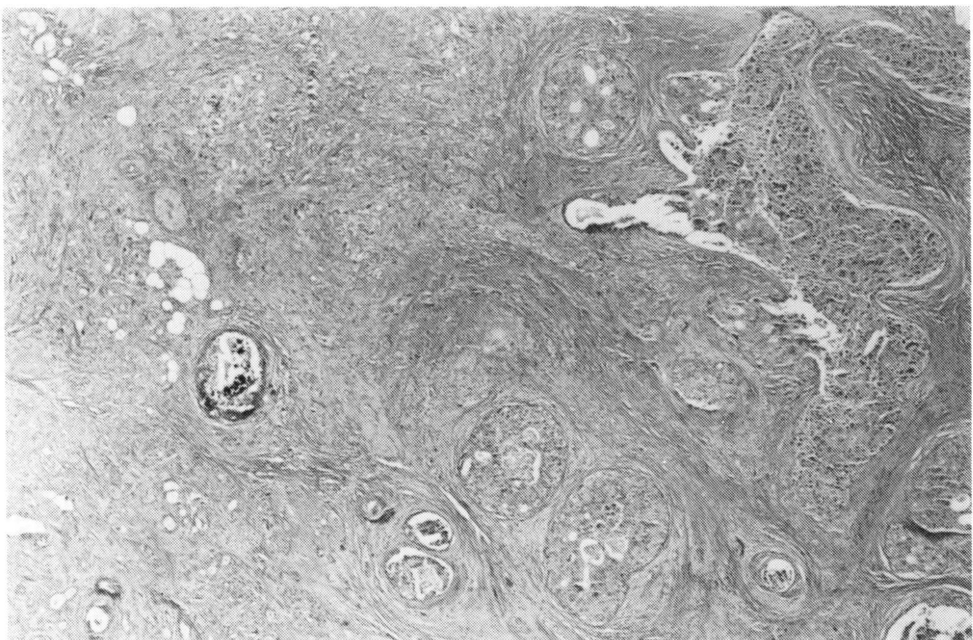

Fig. 3.1A

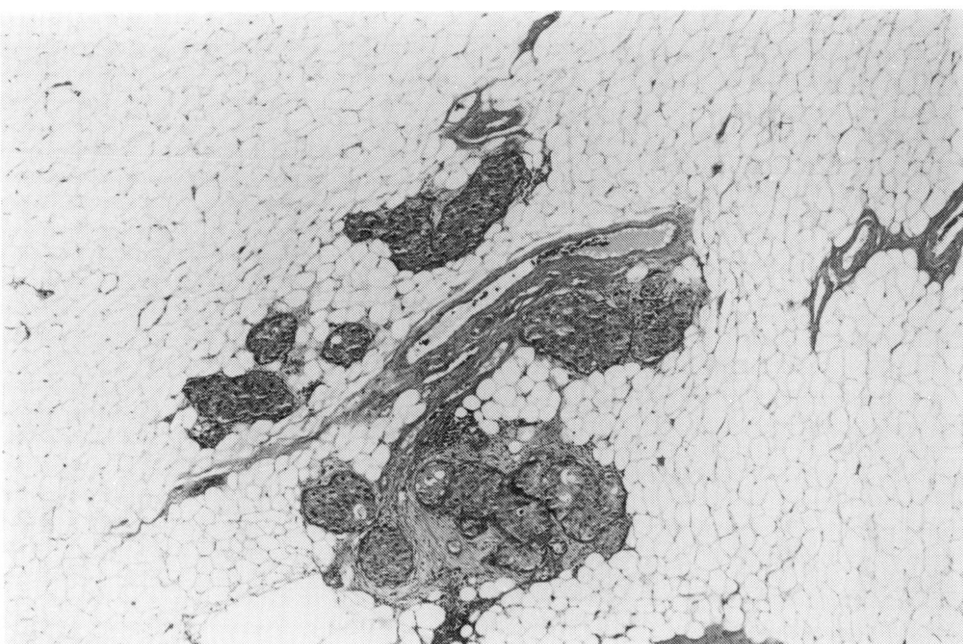

Fig. 3.1B

Fig. 3.1. Extensive intraductal component (EIC) associated with invasive ductal carcinoma. By definition, in EIC the associated intraductal cancer within the tumor constitutes more than 25% of the histological area of the entire tumor mass (Fig. 3.1A). In this 40x photomicrograph, the infiltrating cancer is seen in the upper right and scattered throughout. The intraductal cancer is seen throughout the photomicrograph (especially prominent in the central area) and is quite extensive. EIC also implies extensive intraductal cancer within surrounding normal tissues (40x), as demonstrated in (Fig. 3.1B). Here, an island of fibrous tissue containing ducts involved by intraductal carcinoma is seen in the middle of an area of otherwise uninvolved fatty breast tissue.

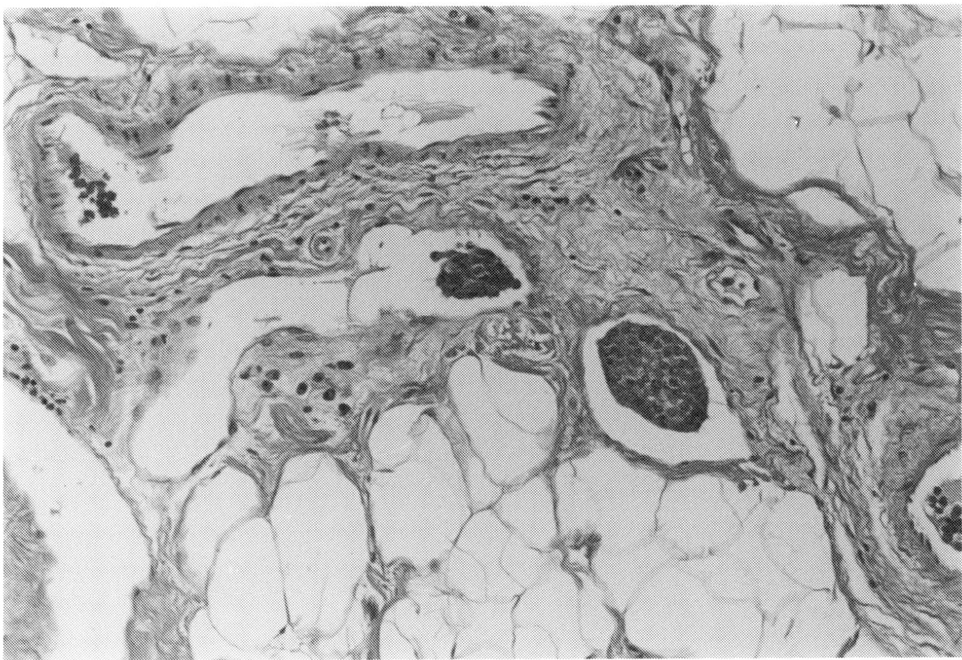

Fig. 3.2. Above: *Lymphatic invasion in the breast tissue surrounding a primary breast cancer. Two large tumor emboli are seen within the thin-walled lymphatic vessels seen in the center of this 200x photomicrograph, with smaller tumor emboli seen superiorly to the left and at the lower right edge of the field.*

Fig. 3.3. Below: *Invasion by breast carcinoma of a vein in the breast tissues adjacent to the primary cancer. The smooth muscle wall of the vein is seen in the center of this 200x photomicrograph, and much of the lumen is filled by tumor.*

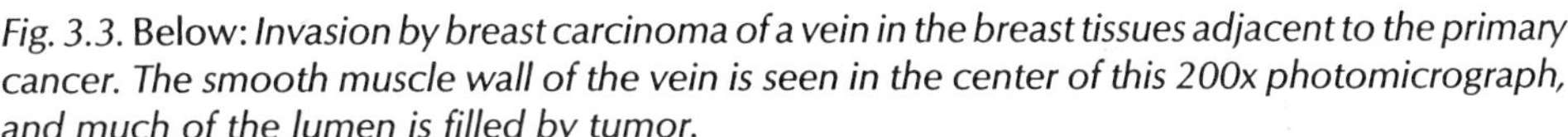

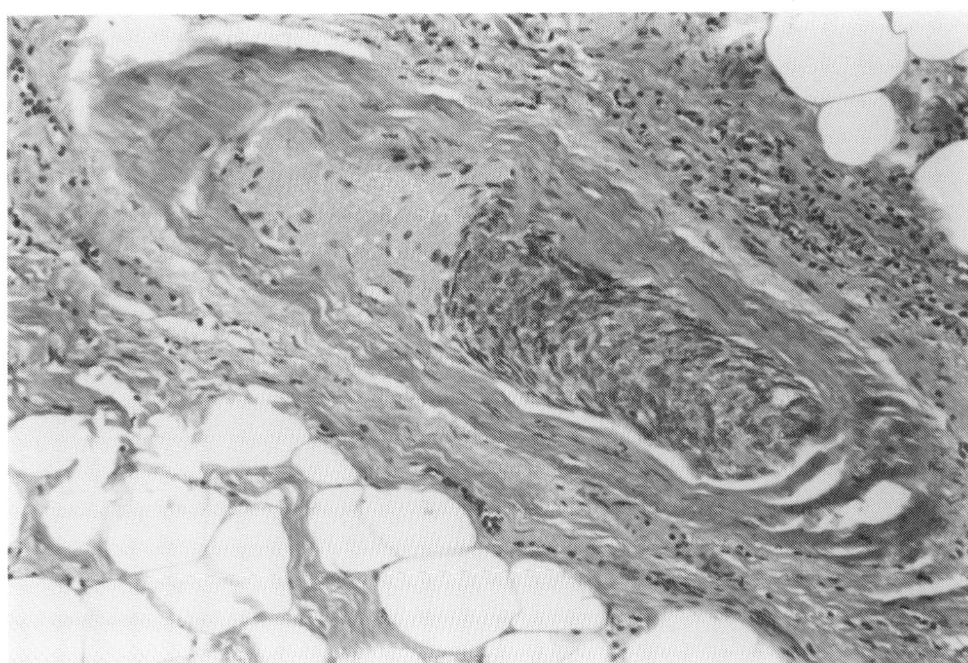

LYMPHATIC OR VASCULAR INVASION WITHIN THE BREAST

Invasion of the lymphatics or veins within the primary tumor and the surrounding breast parenchyma (Fig. 3.2 and 3.3) was found to correlate with multicentricity in the NSABP B-04 study.[57] The five-year analysis of the NSABP B-06 trial revealed that lymphatic or vascular permeation by tumor connoted an excess risk for local recurrence in both of the breast conservation arms.[58] Clemente et al[77] reported similar findings in patients undergoing quadrantectomy, axillary dissection and radiotherapy at the Milan National Cancer Institute. This association has been observed by Fourquet et al,[42,46] Kurtz et al[50] and Vicini et al[71] but was not found in other series.[76,78]

MONONUCLEAR CELL REACTION

Infiltration of mononuclear inflammatory cells into and around the primary breast cancer can be measured semiquantitatively. Intense mononuclear cell reaction (MCR) is an adverse prognostic finding in patients with breast cancer.[48,50] MCR consists mainly of T lymphocytes, and the portion of the infiltrate in direct contact with tumor is made up almost entirely of suppressor T cells. MCR appears to be a histological manifestation of an unfavorable host-tumor relationship. This variable has recently been implicated as a risk factor for local recurrence, especially in younger breast cancer patients.[48,50,53]

AXILLARY NODAL STATUS

Metastatic tumor in the axillary lymph nodes has been reported to be a significant risk factor for tumor relapse in the ipsilateral breast.[40,49,50,78,79] In two of these studies the excess risk was seen only in patients with palpable axillary disease[49,79] and in one series was only demonstrable in postmenopausal patients.[50] However, the NSABP[58,59] and several large retrospective studies[18,47,48,65,80] found no association between local recurrence and axillary nodal status. Haffty et al[45] noted that node-positive patients had a lower incidence of local failure than node-negative patients;

this seemingly paradoxical observation was probably attributable to the use of adjuvant chemotherapy in 88% of the former group.

Patients with axillary nodal metastases are now treated with adjuvant systemic therapy on a routine basis. This is a departure from the recent past; in many of the series demonstrating an excess risk of local failure in node-positive patients, either no adjuvant systemic therapy was administered or the chemotherapy regimen employed was relatively ineffective by modern standards. As noted in chapter 1, adjuvant chemotherapy and tamoxifen probably abrogate the risk of local recurrence; NSABP data suggest that this risk may be lower in node-positive patients treated with adjuvant systemic therapy than in untreated node-negative patients.[15] These data are likely a more accurate reflection of the influence on local recurrence of currently prevailing standards of breast cancer management.

TUMOR HISTOLOGY

Lobular carcinomas were found to have a higher incidence of ipsilateral breast tumor recurrence following breast conservation treatment in one series.[76] Kurtz et al[81] documented a higher frequency of local failure in patients with infiltrating lobular carcinoma, although this trend was not statistically significant. They also noted that recurrences in patients with lobular primaries tended to be multicentric.

In contrast, lobular cancers were not disproportionately multicentric in the NSABP B-04 trial,[82,83] and were not associated with excess risk for local recurrence in the B-06 study.[58] Clarke et al[84] suggested that this apparent discrepancy may be explained by the fact that in the two retrospective studies,[76,81] only gross tumor excision was required whereas in the NSABP B-06 trial, histopathological tumor-free margins of resection were required. Lobular histology may not affect risk of local failure when complete excision of the primary cancer is verified by microscopic examination of the surgical margins.

TUMOR HORMONE RECEPTOR STATUS

Hormone receptor negativity was a significant risk factor in one study[50] and of borderline significance in another retrospective analysis.[85] Hormone receptor status had no significance as a risk factor for local relapse in earlier NSABP analyses[14,58] or in the Princess Margaret Hospital experience.[8] However, more recent results from the NSABP B-06 trial, as presented in Figure 1.1, suggest that estrogen receptor-positive tumors may be less prone to local recurrence.

DNA FLOW CYTOMETRY, ONCOGENES AND OTHER FACTORS

There is an intensive investigative effort underway to elucidate the genetic and molecular events which lead to breast cancer metastasis and mortality. To date, a number of variables have been identified as having prognostic significance in early breast cancer. Among these are DNA flow cytometry parameters,[86-88] tumor cell cytoplasmic cathepsin D content,[89] Pi-class glutathione S-transferase (GST-π) levels in tumor cells,[90] mutant oncogene (*c-myc*,[91] *p53*,[88,92] Nm23,[93] HER-2/ *neu*,[94] etc.) expression, heat shock protein production by tumor cells,[87] and tumor angiogenesis.[95,96] While these have been shown to have prognostic significance as evidenced by their influence on disease-free and overall survival in Stage I breast cancer patients, there are as yet no published data on the predictive value of such variables for local recurrence after breast-conserving treatment.[39]

LOCAL RECURRENCE IN CAREFULLY SELECTED LOW-RISK PATIENTS TREATED BY BREAST-CONSERVING SURGERY WITHOUT RADIOTHERAPY

Adjuvant radiotherapy plays a very important role in breast conservation treatment in that it reduces the chances for tumor recurrence in the ipsilateral breast (Tables 1.4

Table 3.2. Conservative surgery without adjuvant radiotherapy in selected patients at low risk for local recurrence

Institution	No. Patients	Operation*	Selection Criteria	Followup	Ipsilateral Breast Tumor Recurrence Rate	
Uppsala-Örebro Breast Cancer Study Group[97]	192	Sector Resection	• Unifocal tumor ≤ 2 cm. • Microscopic tumor-free margins. • pN– axilla.	3 yrs	7.6%	
Milan National Cancer Institute[98]	273	Quadrantectomy	• Tumor ≤ 2.5 cm. • Microscopic tumor-free margins.	39 mos	8.8%	
University of Miami[74,99]	67	Segmental Mastectomy	• Tumor ≤ 2.5 cm. • Microscopic tumor-free margins ≥ 1 cm. • No EIC • No lymphatic/vascular invasion.	5 yrs	6.4%	
Royal Marsden Hospital[54]	81	Quadrantectomy	• Peripheral tumor ≤ 2 cm. • Microscopic tumor-free margins. • cN– axilla.	5 yrs 5-14 yrs†	10% 11%	
					Stage I	Stage II
Cleveland Clinic[78,100-103]	620	Partial Mastectomy	• Unifocal, peripheral tumor ≤ 2 cm. • Microscopic tumor-free margins. • cN– axilla.	5 yrs 10 yrs	11.1% 14.1%	11.3% 21.6%

cN– clinical node-negative
pN– pathological node-negative

* operations are defined in chapter 1.
† followup period for the entire series.

and 3.1). However, it is apparent from the foregoing discussion that the risk for local recurrence is not uniform among candidates for breast conservation. One of the areas of controversy surrounding ·conservative breast cancer treatment relates to whether combined therapy is necessary for all patients. Are there subsets of patients in whom the risk of local failure is sufficiently small that breast-conserving surgery alone can provide acceptable locoregional control?

The few series in which the incidence of local recurrence following breast-conserving surgery alone was evaluated in carefully selected low-risk patients are summarized in Table 3.2. In all five institutions in which adjuvant radiotherapy has been employed on a selective rather than routine basis, histopathological tumor-free margins of resection have been considered mandatory, especially for patients in whom breast-conserving therapy is limited to surgical excision only.

Two of these studies[97,98] are prospective randomized clinical trials comparing surgery alone to combined therapy. Both demonstrated that patients in the adjuvant radiotherapy arm had fewer breast recurrences than those randomized to surgery only (2.9% versus 7.6% [p = 0.06] in the Uppsala-Örebro trial[97]; 0.3% versus 8.8% [p = 0.001] in the Milan trial[98]). However, it can also be argued that these data show that radiotherapy does not completely eliminate the chance of local failure even in low-risk patients; furthermore, low-risk patients treated by breast-conserving surgery alone do not appear to run a prohibitive risk of ipsilateral breast relapse. The retrospective analyses from three institutions[54,74,78,99-103] cited in Table 3.2 also reported relatively modest local recurrence rates in selected patients treated by breast-conserving surgery alone, as compared to the rates reported in unselected patients (Table 3.1).

The experience of Nemoto et al[18] also provides information relevant to selective use of breast-conserving surgery without radiotherapy. Of their 122 breast cancer patients treated by surgery alone, locoregional recurrences developed in 19% at a median followup of four years. However, none of the

20 patients with tumors less than 1 cm in size failed in the breast, and only one of 31 patients over 70 years of age developed local tumor recurrence.

Thus, it can be argued that combined therapy may not always be necessary whenever breast conservation is undertaken. The risk of ipsilateral breast tumor relapse in some patients may be low enough to permit omission of radiotherapy from their treatment. The proportion of patients which might be eligible for this selective approach is currently unknown, although it probably amounts to no more than a minority, and perhaps a small minority, of breast cancer patients amenable to breast-conserving therapy.

The very modest recurrence rates reported in these series can be attributed at least in part to the care with which surgery was undertaken and submitted tissues were examined. These studies underscore the importance of compulsive attention to detail on the part of both surgeons and pathologists whenever breast-conservation is contemplated. Adjuvant breast irradiation cannot be expected to be effective in the face of sloppy surgery or a cavalier approach to the pathological examination of tissue specimens from the breast and axilla. The surgeon and pathologist share equally in the obligation to ensure that tissue specimens are appropriately oriented, examined grossly and processed properly for histopathology, receptor assays and DNA flow cytometry. Only when all of the relevant pathological information is in hand and its accuracy assured can appropriate recommendations regarding postoperative adjuvant radiation and/or systemic therapy be made.

IPSILATERAL BREAST TUMOR RECURRENCE VERSUS SECOND IPSILATERAL PRIMARY BREAST CANCER

The development of further neoplasia in the conserved breast in the course of followup represents either recurrence (or persistence) of the original primary cancer or presentation of a new tumor which was either occult or not yet present when the original cancer was treated. Time-course studies of ipsilateral breast tumor recurrences following breast-conserving therapy have demonstrated that local treatment failure tends to follow two patterns which fit such a categorization of breast relapses.[7,10,11,36,37,46,66,80,104]

Breast relapses attributed to recurrence of the original primary cancer generally present within the first five to ten years after breast-conserving therapy, develop within or near the site of the original primary cancer (i.e. within the same quadrant of the breast), and are similar or identical to the original cancer in histological appearance.[7,10,21,80,104,105] Haffty et al[80] also used DNA flow cytometric findings as a criterion for distinguishing between true local recurrence and new ipsilateral primary cancer. DNA flow cytometry was deemed to indicate a new primary cancer when the original primary was aneuploid and the relapse diploid. When the original cancer was diploid and the recurrence aneuploid, it could not be concluded that the failure was a new primary as true recurrences are often of a higher grade (and therefore more likely to be aneuploid) than the original cancer.

Recht et al[66] calculated that the hazard rate for true recurrence in the breast climbs over the first 2 1/2 years of followup after breast conservation to 2% per annum and stays at this level until the fifth year, after which it declines to 0.5% per annum by the eighth year (Fig. 3.4). The median interval to recurrence for these lesions was 38.5 months (range: 12 to 87 months). Fowble et al[36] reported a similar disease-free interval for true local recurrences; 65% of breast failures in their series occurred within the vicinity of the original breast cancer, and these constituted 77% of all breast failures presenting within the first five years of followup. Vicini et al[11] and Montague[104] also found that most breast failures occurred near or at the site of the initial lesion. Breast failure presenting as tumor confined to skin, dermis or subcutaneous tissue (that is, outside of the breast parenchyma itself) is by definition recurrence of the original cancer.[7,106]

New metachronous ipsilateral breast cancers are less frequent than true recurrences, and often present years to a decade or more after breast-conserving treatment for the original lesion, although they can occur within the first five years. New ipsilateral cancers frequently develop in sites in the breast remote from the initial cancer, and tend to be histologically distinct from the original tumor. Recht et al[66] noted that the hazard rate for relapses fitting this description increased gradually over the first five years of followup to 1% per annum, and then

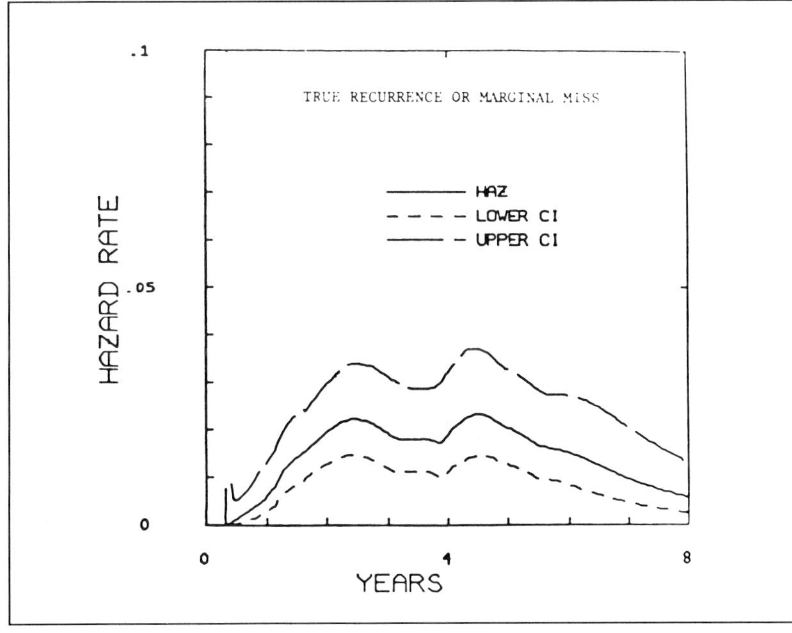

Fig. 3.4. Hazard rate for recurrence at or near the site of the original primary cancer within the conserved breast, as a function of time. These true local recurrences usually develop within the first five years of followup, as shown in this hazard function. Reproduced from Recht A, et al. Int J Radiat Oncol Biol Phys 1988; 15:255-261; © 1988 with kind permission from Elsevier Science Ltd., The Boulevard, Langford Lane, Kidlington OX5 1GB, U.K.

Fig. 3.5. Hazard rate as a function of time for failure at sites in the ipsilateral breast other than that of the original primary carcinoma. These are largely new primary lesions; the hazard rises gradually over the first five years of followup and persists over the long term. Reproduced with permission from Recht A, et al. Int J Radiat Oncol Biol Phys 1988; 15:255-261; © 1988 with kind permission from Elsevier Science Ltd., The Boulevard, Langford Lane, Kidlington OX5 1GB, U.K.

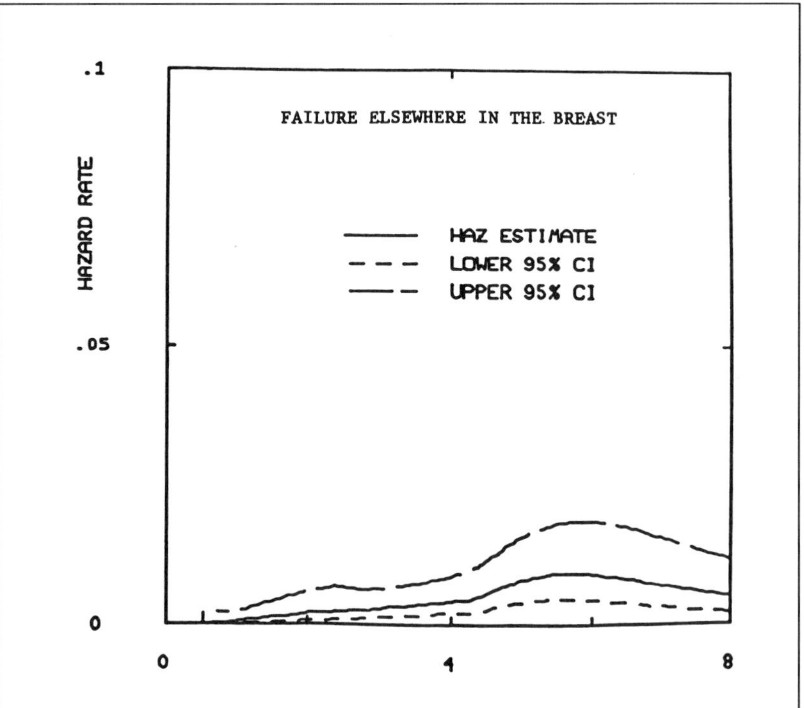

stayed at this level thereafter (Fig. 3.5). The hazard over time for new ipsilateral primary breast cancer in patients treated by breast conservation therefore parallels that for metachronous contralateral breast cancer.

In the experience of Fowble et al,[36] as the time interval to breast relapse increased, the proportion of recurrences which arose in remote sites in the breast also increased; 54% of relapses presenting more than five years after breast-conserving therapy were far removed from the original lumpectomy site. They also noted a predilection for new ipsilateral primary cancers among women aged 35 years or less at the time of primary treatment. Kurtz et al[7] noted that, as compared to breast cancer events within the first five years, late breast tumor recurrences were less frequently inoperable (1.4% versus 17%), more often distant from the original primary, and had a significantly better prognosis. The risk for new ipsilateral breast cancer was only appreciable after five years, but in the second decade of followup these lesions constituted the majority of local failures.

The interval to recurrence has been correlated with the location of the breast recurrence with respect to the site of the original primary cancer.[105] Of all ipsilateral breast tumor recurrences in this series, 90% presenting within two years of initial breast-conserving therapy were in the vicinity of the original primary. In the course of subsequent followup the proportion of relapses near or within the original primary site was 83% for recurrences presenting 3 to 7 years after initial treatment, 68% for those diagnosed at 8 to 10 years followup, and 45% at 11 to 15 years. All three ipsilateral breast failures during or after the sixteenth year of followup developed in remote sites in the breast.

THE BIOLOGICAL SIGNIFICANCE OF LOCAL RECURRENCE

LOCAL RECURRENCE FOLLOWING RADICAL SURGERY

In patients who have undergone curative radical or modified radical mastectomy, recurrence of tumor within the mastectomy

Table 3.3. Overall and disease-free survival in patients with isolated local recurrence following radical breast cancer surgery

Series	No. Patients with Local Recurrence	Overall Survival*			Disease-free Survival*		
		3 yrs	5 yrs	10 yrs	3 yrs	5 yrs	10 yrs
Auchincloss[107]	22	23%	14%	—	—	—	—
Gilliland[108]	60	—	18%	5%	—	—	—
Toonkel[109]	121	—	38%	26%	—	26%	15%
Aberizk[110]	90	—	50%	26%	—	30%	7%
Deutsch[111]	107	—	35%	—	—	—	—
Chu[112]	215	—	21%	5%	—	24%	—
Schwaibold[113]	128	—	49%	—	—	24%	—
Beck[114]	121	—	—	22%	—	—	12%
Dao[115]	13	31%	—	—	8%	—	—
Donegan[116]	146	15%	4%	0%	—	—	—
Stadler[117]	134	—	22%	—	—	—	—
Bedwinek[118]	129	—	36%	—	—	13%	—
Zimmerman[119]	203	—	3%	—	—	—	—
Fentiman[120]	73	44%	30%	12%	15%	4%	—
Halverson[121]	224	—	43%	26%	—	26%	15%

* After treatment of local recurrence.

scar, skin flaps or chest wall as a first breast cancer event is an ominous development. The vast majority of affected patients will die of disseminated breast cancer within ten years of treatment of the local tumor relapse. Table 3.3 summarizes data pertinent to the prognosis of local recurrence following radical surgery for breast cancer.

Locoregional recurrence after radical or modified radical mastectomy usually portends a fatal outcome. At least 80% of affected patients will succumb to disseminated breast cancer, most within two to three years of the local recurrence. In the series of Gilliland et al,[108] all patients with postmastectomy local recurrence ultimately died of metastatic breast cancer.

Karabali-Dalamaga et al[122] observed that in patients in whom locoregional disease was the first and only sign of relapse, time intervals to recurrence followed an exponential curve which was superimposable on that of patients in whom distant metastasis was the first sign of breast cancer relapse. Postrelapse survival was only modestly (albeit significantly) better for those whose first recurrence was locoregional rather than distant, with

approximately 90% actuarial mortality at seven years. Adjuvant radiotherapy following mastectomy did not delay the onset of locoregional recurrence in this series. The rate of appearance of distant metastases following locoregional recurrence was about 20% per year in the series of Aberizk et al.[110] Greco et al[123] observed that the prognostic significance of first recurrence in the mastectomy scar or flaps was essentially the same as that of distant dermal or subcutaneous metastases.

A short disease-free interval from time of initial surgery to recurrence,[109-111,113,123] multiple nodules or larger recurrence as compared to a single focus or limited area of recurrent cancer,[113,123] simultaneous chest wall and regional nodal recurrence,[109,111] and persistence or further locoregional relapse after salvage treatment for the initial recurrence[108,112,113] signify a particularly poor prognosis.

Much of the early resistance to breast conservation therapy within the medical profession was based on the overwhelming incidence of breast cancer mortality associated with local recurrence following radical surgery. There was concern that conservative locoregional treatment might eventuate in much more frequent locoregional disease recurrence, which in turn would lead to higher breast cancer death rates than mastectomy. In essence, the association between locoregional recurrence and systemic dissemination of breast cancer after radical or modified radical mastectomy was deemed by many to be causal.

Local Recurrence Following Breast-Conserving Therapy

The first reports of limited surgery and radiotherapy for early breast cancer provided some assurance that locoregional recurrence following breast conservation does not have the dire significance of local failure after mastectomy.[100,124,125] Several subsequent nonrandomized studies[5,8,47,85,101,102,126-128] corroborated this observation.

The prospective randomized studies reviewed in chapter 1 examined the effect of ipsilateral breast tumor recurrence on prognosis. The NSABP B-06 trial results at five years'[12] and eight years'[13] followup suggested that local recurrence after segmental mastectomy with or without breast radiotherapy had no effect on long term survival. The findings of the U.S. National Cancer Institute trial[3] corroborated those of NSABP B-06. The outcomes of the Milan study[106,129-131] of radical mastectomy versus quadrantectomy, axillary lymphadenectomy and radiotherapy and a subsequent trial of lumpectomy plus radiation versus quadrantectomy plus radiation[132] also suggested that local failure had no influence on long term outcome. Thus, it was proposed that tumor relapse in the treated breast following conservative management does not prejudice the prospects for long term cure in affected patients.

However, some studies of breast conservation suggested that patients with local recurrence were more likely to die of disseminated breast cancer than those who did not recur. The EORTC 10801 trial[1] comparing modified radical mastectomy to breast conservation reported that postsalvage survival of patients who developed local recurrence was identical for both treatment arms. Chauvet et al[6] found that patients with local tumor recurrence were significantly more likely to develop distant metastases and die of breast cancer. Osborne et al[79] reported only 50% overall survival and 42% relapse-free survival five years after local recurrence in their series. Leung et al[60] found only 23 of

Table 3.4. Overall and disease-free survival* in patients with local recurrence following conservative surgery and radiotherapy for early breast cancer

Series	No. Patients with Local Recurrence	Overall Survival		Disease-free Survival	
		5 yrs	10 yrs	5 yrs	10 yrs
Calle[5]	21	–	–	87%	75%
Chauvet[6]	16	88%	–	80%	–
Recht[10]	30	54%	–	43%	–
	16 resectable	68%	–	54%	–
Harris[21]	30	–	–	58%	50%
Fowble[36]	65	84%	–	59%	–
Fourquet[45]	56	73%	–	–	–
Kurtz[105]	171	69%	57%	–	–
Haffty[133]	38	–	–	54%	–
Stotter[134]	49	79%	64%	–	–
Spitalier[135]	96	61%	–	–	–
Abner[136]	123	79%	–	56%	–
Kurtz[137]	118	72%	58%	–	–
Osborne[138]	46	76%	–	55%	–
Cajucom[139]	25	65%	–	51%	–

* Post-reoccurance survival

45 patients to be free of disease three years after treatment for locoregional failure; six of these local recurrences had been unresectable at the time of presentation. The excess risk of mortality posed by local recurrence in most of these studies was smaller than that associated with local relapse following radical surgery, but was nonetheless a worrisome finding. Postrelapse survival data from retrospective studies of breast-conserving therapy are given in Table 3.4.

In an attempt to address the controversy surrounding the significance of locoregional relapse after breast conservation, Stotter et al[134] postulated that locoregional recurrence following breast-conserving therapy may be associated with an excess survival hazard comparable to that of a second primary cancer. Using a mathematical model, they predicted a postrecurrence five-year survival of 61%; this figure would be 83% if local recurrence connoted no excess risk for mortality. The actuarial survival of 49 patients with locoregional recurrence (of 449 patients treated with breast-conserving therapy) was used to test this hypothesis. The observed five-year postrecurrence survival was 63%.

The authors concluded that local recurrence is associated with a modest excess risk of breast cancer mortality. However, this excess risk was felt to be so small that at least 10,000 patients followed prospectively for a minimum of 10 years would be required to detect it. It was suggested that the NSAB-B06 and Milan trials had insufficient numbers of patients to detect any association between local recurrence and risk of mortality.

After a followup period of nine years, the NSABP B-06 trial was re-analyzed, this time with the added intent of addressing the prognostic implications of local relapse following breast conservation.[14,15] Hazard rates were estimated by a Cox proportional hazards model with adjustment for twelve covariates, the selection of which was based on data from previous NSABP studies. Ipsilateral breast tumor recurrence was found to be a highly significant predictor of development of distant metastases with a relative risk of 3.41 as compared to patients in whom breast tumor relapse did not occur.

At nine years followup, 43% of the B-06 patients treated by segmental mastectomy

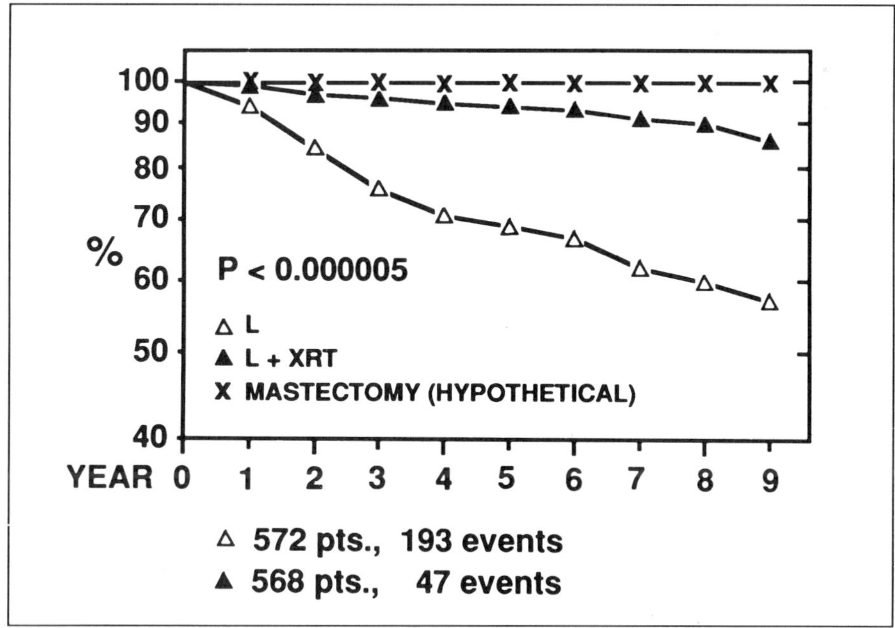

Fig. 3.6. Ipsilateral breast tumor recurrence following segmental mastectomy with or without breast irradiation in the NSABP B-06 trial. Reproduced with permission of Wiley-Liss, a Division of John Wiley and Sons, Inc.; from Fisher B, et al. Semin Surg Oncol 1992; 8:153-160, ©1992.

only had relapsed in the breast as compared to 12% of patients treated by segmental mastectomy and breast irradiation (Fig. 3.6). Despite this highly significant difference in incidence of breast recurrence, there were no differences between these two groups or between either group and the patients in the total mastectomy arm in terms of disease-free, distant disease-free or overall survival. Abrogation of the risk of local relapse by adjuvant radiotherapy or total mastectomy did not alter the underlying long-term risk of disseminated disease.

Therefore, it was concluded that ipsilateral breast tumor relapse is not causally related to distant metastasis and breast cancer death, but is simply a marker of increased risk for these events. Ablation of the marker by mastectomy or radiotherapy does not change the underlying risk for breast cancer metastasis and mortality. This conclusion is analogous to that reached in the NSABP B-04 trial regarding the significance of axillary nodal involvement, in which it was established that axillary metastases are "indicators", and not "instigators", of breast cancer dissemination.[14]

Factors Predictive of Poor Prognosis in Patients with Local Relapse after Breast-Conserving Therapy

A number of factors which portend a poor outcome have been identified in patients with ipsilateral locoregional recurrence after conservative breast cancer treatment. Approximately 10% of locoregional recurrences are accompanied by the simultaneous development of distant metastases, and 5% to 15% are unresectable at the time they are detected;[7,36,85,105,135,140] survival of affected patients is much worse than that of patients with isolated, operable recurrence.[60,79,85,105,141,142]

Patients with large, extensive or diffuse local recurrences following breast conservation treatment have a more guarded outlook than those in whom the recurrence is small (less than 2 to 3 cm) or limited in extent.[4,36,47,105,139,143,144] Similarly, those with simultaneous breast and regional nodal relapse or nodal relapse alone fare worse than

those with isolated breast failure.[7,9,47,140] Cajucom et al[139] found that patients in whom more than four positive axillary nodes were resected at the time of locoregional relapse had a much worse prognosis than those with three or fewer involved nodes. Dermal recurrence also connotes a much higher probability of breast cancer mortality.[4,47]

The time interval from breast-conservation therapy for the primary breast cancer to detection of local recurrence as a first breast cancer event has prognostic significance. Recurrence within the first two years following breast-conserving therapy was found to be predictive of an adverse outcome in several series.[4,46,105,141,145] Chauvet et al[145] found that postrelapse survival of patients with local recurrence within two years of initial surgery was only 39.5% as compared to 80.5% of patients with a longer disease-free interval to recurrence. On the other hand, patients with late ipsilateral breast tumor recurrences were more likely to have a benign postrelapse clinical course; Kurtz et al[141] suggested that local tumor recurrences five or more years after initial treatment were analogous to second contralateral breast cancers in terms of their prognostic significance. Haffty et al[80] noted that patients who developed a true local recurrence had an actuarial five-year survival of only 39% as compared to 89% (p < 0.05) for patients in whom breast relapse was considered to be a new ipsilateral primary cancer. Median interval to breast relapse was 3.2 years in the former group and 5.4 years in the latter (p < 0.05).

As already noted, most true local recurrences develop within the first five years after conservative treatment and are found within or close to the segmental mastectomy site, or at least within the same quadrant of the breast as the original primary. Relapse in the ipsilateral breast in a site remote from the original primary cancer is associated with a better prognosis overall.[4,7,80]

The histology of the breast recurrence has been found to be of prognostic significance in some series. Abner et al[136] and Recht et al[140] reported that patients with in situ or microinvasive recurrences fared significantly better in subsequent followup than those with predominantly invasive relapses. Chauvet et al[145] noted that patients in whom the recurrent disease had a smaller proportion of noninvasive carcinoma than the initial primary cancer had a higher incidence of metastasis and disease-specific mortality (52.5% versus 93.3% two-year survival postrecurrence) than those in whom in situ disease was present in the same proportion as in the original cancer.

The stage of the original tumor at the time of initial conservative management is also a significant predictor of behavior of disease after first locoregional relapse.[144] Barr et al[9] reported uncontrolled local or nodal recurrence in 7 of 356 (2%) Stage I and II breast cancers and in 9 of 55 patients (16%) with Stage III and IV disease at initial diagnosis. Eight of the nine patients with advanced stage tumor and uncontrollable locoregional recurrence died of their disease. Spitalier et al[135] found that postrelapse survival prospects were more favorable in Stage I breast cancer patients, although the risk of locoregional relapse developing was no higher in Stage II than Stage I disease. Kurtz et al[137] noted that Stage I patients with local recurrence had a favorable prognosis irrespective of the interval to breast relapse.

Haffty et al[133] studied the prognostic significance of DNA flow cytometry of recurrent cancer in the ipsilateral breast in 50 patients. In multivariate analysis, tumor cell ploidy was a significant independent prognostic indicator of postrecurrence disease-free survival. Patients with diploid recurrences had a five-year survival rate of 64% as compared to 15% for aneuploid recurrences (p = 0.02). Five-year survival was 83% for patients in whom the S-phase fraction (SPF) of the recurrent disease was less than 12%, as compared to 24% survival among those in whom SPF was 12% or greater. "Favorable" recurrences (those which were diploid with SPF < 12%) were associated with an 89% five-year overall survival and 100% disease-free survival, as compared to "unfavorable" (aneuploid with SPF ≥ 12%) relapses, which had a 24% overall and 32% disease-free survival (p = 0.01).

SALVAGE OF IPSILATERAL BREAST TUMOR RECURRENCE

The NSABP B-06 trial stipulated that ipsilateral breast tumor recurrence in study participants be treated by completion total mastectomy whenever surgical resection was possible.[12-16] This policy reflected the preferred routine management of local recurrence in centers in which breast conservation was being used at the time the B-06 trial protocol was written.

In patients treated by breast conservation, ipsilateral breast tumor relapse can effectively be managed by completion total mastectomy with a low risk of complications. The documented incidence of second local recurrence after salvage mastectomy ranges from 4% to 32%, with most series reporting second local failures in less than 15% of patients.[7,8,36,137-141,146,147]

In patients with initially inoperable breast tumor recurrences, the use of preoperative adjuvant chemotherapy has been used with success to obtain a partial response, thereby making the recurrence amenable to resection by completion mastectomy.[6,147]

It has been postulated that not all ipsilateral breast failures require total mastectomy for excellent local control. A number of centers have resorted to a second breast-conserving operation for salvage in selected patients.[4,7-9,40,105,127,135,137,141,142,146-148] Fowble et al[36] investigated whether completion total mastectomy is always necessary by examining mastectomy specimens from 31 patients in whom complete gross excision of the recurrent disease had been performed for diagnosis of local failure prior to "definitive" surgery. There was no residual tumor in 13 completion mastectomy specimens (42%); the absence of residual cancer correlated with age over 35 years, negative or unknown axillary nodal status, categorization of the breast relapse as a true recurrence of the original primary cancer and little or no associated intraductal disease. Half of the remaining total mastectomies harbored residual cancer in two or more quadrants of the breast.

The proportion of ipsilateral breast tumor recurrences amenable to secondary breast-conserving surgery has varied somewhat between series. Patients who refuse completion total mastectomy may be offered this option,[4,140] and those in whom treatment of the original primary consisted of breast-conserving surgery without adjuvant radiotherapy can often be offered a second conservative excision with breast irradiation postoperatively.[8,148]

In general, secondary breast-conserving surgery has been performed in patients with small, slowly growing recurrences.[7,9,60,105,127,135,137,141,146] Kurtz et al[137,146] considered that conservative salvage surgery for ipsilateral breast tumor relapse was warranted only for recurrences of 2 cm or less in diameter with no fixation to skin or chest wall, and no tumor-related erythema, edema or other signs of rapid growth. In addition, they restricted the use of conservative salvage surgery to patients with node-negative cancer in whom there was little or no chronic radiation change (fibrosis, retraction, telangiectasia, etc.) in the affected breast. When conservative surgery was used in 52 patients with recurrence who met these criteria, there were 12 subsequent (i.e. second) breast failures (23%) at a median postrecurrence interval of 36 months. Two of these were inoperable while the other 10 were treated with further surgery. This compares to a 12% incidence of second recurrence among 66 patients in whom the first local relapse was managed by completion mastectomy; these patients had more extensive recurrences than those whose breast failures were managed by conservative salvage surgery.

In a retrospective time-course study of ipsilateral breast tumor recurrence, Kurtz et al[105] found that postrecurrence survival was not affected by the type of salvage surgery used to treat the breast failure. However, patients whose local recurrences were managed by breast-conserving surgery had a 36% five-year actuarial incidence of second breast recurrence as compared to a 12% incidence among those undergoing salvage mastectomy. This discrepancy in incidence of second local failure in favor of mastectomy was seen even though the mastectomy-treated patients had more extensive first recurrences. In a study

of late first local relapses, Kurtz et al[7] using the same criteria for conservative salvage surgery reported five-year postrecurrence local control rates of 86% and 96% for first recurrences treated by breast-conservation and completion mastectomy, respectively. There was no significant difference in disease-free survival related to the type of surgical salvage procedure used. Completion mastectomy is probably superior to conservative salvage surgery in terms of control of the breast failure, but a second attempt at breast salvage when local recurrence develops is often successful in appropriately selected patients, and is not prejudicial to postrecurrence survival.

McCready et al[148] reported their experience with surgical salvage of breast relapse in patients initially treated by conservative surgery without radiotherapy. Tumor-free margins were histologically confirmed in all patients in whom the surgical salvage procedure was conservative. Nineteen patients in whom ipsilateral breast tumor relapse was treated by a second breast-conserving operation plus adjuvant breast radiotherapy had a five-year actuarial postrecurrence local recurrence rate of 18%. Twenty-seven patients with breast tumor relapses treated by repeat breast-conserving surgery alone had a 68% local failure rate. Given that the size of recurrence was essentially the same for both groups, the efficacy of the addition of breast irradiation to conservative salvage surgery in these clinical circumstances is readily apparent.

COMPLICATIONS OF SALVAGE SURGERY FOR LOCAL RECURRENCE

As breast conservation treatment includes the use of both surgery and adjuvant radiotherapy, there has been some concern about possible morbidity related to the use of salvage surgery in the irradiated field. In general, the complication rate has proven to be quite low[142] and the aesthetic outcome of conservative salvage surgery acceptable when there are only minimal to mild chronic radiation changes evident in the conserved breast.[137,146]

Stotter et al[147] noted complications in 26% of patients undergoing salvage surgery for local recurrence. These included wound infection, delayed healing and flap necrosis.

However, most of these were minor, and did not greatly affect postoperative convalescence of the affected patients. Leung et al[60] reported delayed wound healing in a small number of their 45 surgically salvageable patients, only one of which was significant. Osborne et al[138] reported a complication rate of 7%, which was comparable to that seen in nonirradiated breast cancer patients. Complications included one wound infection, one hematoma and one flap necrosis among their 46 patients.

ADJUVANT SYSTEMIC THERAPY FOLLOWING SALVAGE SURGERY FOR IPSILATERAL BREAST TUMOR RECURRENCE

Having confirmed the significance of ipsilateral breast tumor relapse as a marker of risk for breast cancer dissemination, Fisher et al[14,16] suggested that adjuvant systemic therapy should be tested in future randomized trials in patients with local recurrence following breast-conserving therapy to evaluate whether the increased risk for metastasis can be abrogated. Several retrospective studies have included patients treated with adjuvant chemotherapy for local recurrence, either before or after salvage surgery.[6,8,36,136,139,147] Chemotherapy has been administered to these patients either to facilitate the resectability of the recurrence, or in recognition of the increased future risk for metastatic breast cancer.

To date, the use of adjuvant chemotherapy in this clinical setting has not been shown to be of significant benefit. A large number of patients will have to be studied in a multicenter prospective randomized trial to determine whether systemic chemotherapy can reduce the risk of breast cancer mortality among patients with locoregional recurrence following breast-conserving therapy.

REFERENCES

1. Van Dongen JA, Bartelink H, Fentiman IS, et al. Randomized clinical trial to assess the value of breast-conserving therapy in Stage I and II breast cancer, EORTC 10801 trial. J Natl Cancer Inst Monogr 1992; 11:15-18.
2. Blichert-Toft M, Rose C, Andersen JA, et al. Danish randomized trial comparing breast conservation therapy with mas-tectomy: six years of life-table analysis. J Natl Cancer Inst Monogr 1992; 11:19-26.
3. Straus K, Lichter A, Lippman M, et al. Results of the National Cancer Institute Early Breast Cancer Trial. J Natl Cancer Inst Monogr 1992; 11:27-31.
4. Haffty BG, Goldberg NB, Fischer D, et al. Conservative surgery and radiation therapy in breast carcinoma: local recurrence and prognostic implications. Int J Radiat Oncol Biol Phys 1989; 17:727-732.
5. Calle R, Vilcoq JR, Zafrani B, Vielh P, Fourquet A. Local control and survival of breast cancer treated by limited surgery followed by irradiation. Int J Radiat Oncol Biol Phys 1986; 12:873-878.
6. Chauvet B, Reynaud-Bougnoux A, Calais G, et al. Prognostic significance of breast relapse after conservative treatment in node-negative early breast cancer. Int J Radiat Oncol Biol Phys 1990; 19:1125-1130.
7. Kurtz JM, Spitalier J-M, Amalric R, et al. The prognostic significance of late local recurrence after breast-conserving therapy. Int J Radiat Oncol Biol Phys 1990; 19:87-93.
8. Clark RM, Wilkinson RH, Miceli PN, MacDonald WD. Breast Cancer. Experiences with conservation therapy. Amer J Clin Oncol 1987; 10:461-468.
9. Barr LC, Brunt AM, Goodman AG, Phillips RH, Ellis H. Uncontrolled local recurrence after treatment of breast cancer with breast conservation. Cancer 1989; 64:1203-1207.
10. Recht A, Silver B, Schnitt S, et al. Breast relapse following primary radiation therapy for early breast cancer. I. Classification, frequency, and salvage. Int J Radiat Oncol Biol Phys 1985; 11:1271-1276.
11. Vicini FA, Recht A, Abner A, et al. Recurrence in the breast following conservative surgery and radiation therapy for early stage breast cancer. J Natl Cancer Inst Monogr 1992; 11:33-40.
12. Fisher B, Bauer M, Margolese R, et al. Five-year results of a randomized clinical trial comparing total mastectomy and segmental mastectomy with or without radiation in the treatment of breast cancer. New Engl J Med 1985; 312:665-673.
13. Fisher B, Redmond C, Poisson R, et al. Eight-year results of a randomized clinical trial com-

paring total mastectomy and lumpectomy with or without irradiation in the treatment of breast cancer. New Engl J Med 1989; 320:822-828.

14. Fisher B, Anderson S, Fisher ER, et al. Significance of ipsilateral breast tumour recurrence after lumpectomy. Lancet 1991; 338:327-331.

15. Fisher B, Redmond C, and other NSABP investigators. Lumpectomy for breast cancer: an update of the NSABP experience. J Natl Cancer Inst Monogr 1992; 11:7-14.

16. Fisher B, Wickerham DL, Deutsch M, et al. Breast tumor recurrence following lumpectomy with or without breast irradiation: an overview of recent NSABP findings. Semin Surg Oncol 1992; 8:153-160.

17. Hallahan DE, Michel AG, Halpern HJ, et al. Breast conserving surgery and definitive irradiation for early stage breast cancer. Int J Radiat Oncol Biol Phys 1989; 17: 1211-1216.

18. Nemoto T, Patel JK, Rosner D, et al. Factors affecting recurrence in lumpectomy without irradiation for breast cancer. Cancer 1991; 67:2079-2082.

19. Lagios MD, Richards VE, Rose ME, Yee E. Segmental mastectomy without radiotherapy: short-term followup. Cancer 1983; 52: 2173-2179.

20. Montgomery ACV, Greening WP, Levene AL. Clinical study of recurrence rate and survival time of patients with carcinoma of the breast treated by biopsy excision without any other therapy. J Roy Soc Med 1978; 71:339-342.

21. Harris JR, Recht A, Amalric R, et al. Time course and prognosis of local recurrence following primary radiation therapy for early breast cancer. J Clin Oncol 1984; 2:37-41.

22. Beadle GF, Silver B, Botnick L, Hellman S, Harris JR. Cosmetic results following primary radiation therapy for early breast cancer. Cancer 1984; 54:2911-2918.

23. Clarke D, Martinez A, Coe RS, Goffinet DR. Breast edema following staging axillary dissection in patients with bresat carcinoma treated by radical radiotherapy. Cancer 1982; 49:2295-2299.

24. Clarke D, Martinez A, Cox RS. Analysis of cosmetic results and complications in patients with Stage I and II breast cancer treated by

biopsy and irradiation. Int J Radiat Oncol Biol Phys 1983; 9:1807-1813.

25. Bostwick J, Paletta C, Hartrampf CR. Conservative treatment for breast cancer. Complications requiring reconstructive surgery. Ann Surg 1986; 203:481-490.

26. Welch JS. The postirradiated breast. Mayo Clin Proc 1986; 61:392-395.

27. Clarke D, Curtis JL, Martinez A, et al. Fat necrosis of the breast simulating recurrent carcinoma after primary radiotherapy in the management of early stage breast carcinoma. Cancer 1983; 52:442-445.

28. Lipsztein R, Dalton JF, Bloomer WD. Sequelae of breast irradiation. J Amer Med Assoc 1985; 253:3582-3584.

29. El-Deeb NA. Fat necrosis of the breast: an unusual complication of lumpectomy and radiotherapy in breast cancer. Review of the literature and report of four new cases. Eur J Surg Oncol 1990; 16:248-250.

30. Pezner RD, Lorant JA, Terz J, et al. Wound-healing complications following biopsy of the irradiated breast. Arch Surg 1992; 127:321-324.

31. Solin SJ, Fowble BL, Schultz DJ, Rubenstein JR, Goodman RL. The detection of local recurrence after definitive irradiation for early stage carcinoma of the breast. Cancer 1990; 65:2497-2502.

32. Sickles EA, Ominsky SH, Sollitto RA, Galvin HB, Monticicciolo DL. Medical audit of rapid-throughput mammography screening practice: methodology and results of 27,114 examinations. Radiology 1990; 175:323-327.

33. Dershaw DD, Shank B, Reisinger S. Mammographic findings following breast cancer treatment by local excision and definitive irradiation. Radiology 1987; 164:455-461.

34. Dershaw DD, McCormick B, Cox L, Osborne MP. Benign and malignant tumor recurrence at the surgical site after conservative therapy for breast carcinoma. Amer J Roentgenol 1990; 155:35-38.

35. Stomper PC, Recht A, Berenberg AL, Tochelson MS, Harris JR. Mammographic detection of recurrent cancer in the irradiated breast. Amer J Roentgenol 1987; 143:39-43.

36. Fowble B, Solin LJ, Schultz DJ, et al. Breast recurrence following conservative surgery and radiation: patterns of failure, prognosis, and

pathologic findings from mastectomy specimens with implications for treatment. Int J Radiat Oncol Biol Phys 1990; 19:833-842.

37. Schnitt SJ, Connolly JL, Recht A, Silver B, Harris JR. Breast relapse following primary radiation therapy for early breast cancer. II. Detection, pathologic features and prognostic significance. Int J Radiat Oncol Biol Phys 1985; 11:1277-1284.

38. Dershaw DD, McCormick B, Osborne MP. Detection of local recurrence after conservative therapy for breast carcinoma. Cancer 1992; 70:493-496.

39. Kurtz JM. Factors influencing the risk of local recurrence in the breast. Eur J Cancer 1992; 28:660-666.

40. Delouche G, Bachelot F, Premont M, Kurtz JM. Conservation treatment of early breast cancer: long term results and complications. Int J Radiat Oncol Biol Phys 1987; 13:29-34.

41. Bartelink H, Borger JH, van Dongen JA, Peterse JL. The impact of tumor size and histology on local control after breast-conserving therapy. Radiother Oncol 1988; 11: 297-303.

42. Fourquet A, Vilcoq JR, Zafrani B, Durand JC, Mosseri V. Early stage breast cancer: a multivariate analysis of the risk of local recurrence following conservative treatment. Long term results. Int J Radiat Oncol Biol Phys 1988; 15(Suppl 1):181 (Abstr).

43. Boyages J, Recht A, Connolly JL, et al. Factors associated with local recurrence as a first site of failure following the conservative treatment of early breast cancer. Int J Radiat Oncol Biol Phys 1986; 12 (Suppl 1):93 (Abstr).

44. Vilcoq JR, Calle R, Stacey P, Ghossein NA. The outcome of treatment by tumorectomy and radiotherapy of patients with operable breast cancer. Int J Radiat Oncol Biol Phys 1981; 7:1327-1332.

45. Haffty BG, Fischer D, Rose M, Beinfeld M, McKhann C. Prognostic factors for local recurrence in the conservatively treated breast cancer patient: a cautious interpretation of the data. J Clin Oncol 1991; 9:997-1003.

46. Fourquet A, Campana F, Zafrani B, et al. Prognostic factors of breast recurrence in the conservative management of early breast cancer: a 25-year followup. Int J Radiat Oncol Biol Phys 1989; 17:719-725.

47. Clarke DH, Lê MG, Sarrazin D, et al. Analysis of local-regional relapses in patients with early breast cancers treated by excision and radiotherapy: experience of the Institut Gustave-Roussy. Int J Radiat Oncol Biol Phys 1985; 11:137-145.

48. Kurtz JM, Jacquemier J, Amalric R, et al. Why are local recurrences after breast-conserving therapy more frequent in younger patients? J Clin Oncol 1990; 8:591-598.

49. Van Limbergen E, van den Bogaert W, van der Schueren E, Rijnders A. Tumor excision and radiotherapy as primary treatment of breast cancer. Analysis of patient and treatment parameters and local control. Radiother Oncol 1987; 8:1-9.

50. Kurtz JM, Jacquemier J, Amalric R, et al. Risk factors for breast recurrence in premenopausal and postmenopausal patients with ductal cancers treated by conservation therapy. Cancer 1990; 65:1867-1878.

51. Peterse JL, van Dongen JA, Bartelink H. Recurrence of breast carcinoma after breast-conserving therapy. Eur J Surg Oncol 1988; 14:123-126.

52. Recht A, Connolly JL, Schnitt SJ, Silver B, Harris JR. Conservative surgery and radiotherapy for early breast cancer: the effect of age on breast recurrence. Int J Radiat Oncol Biol Phys 1986; 12(Suppl 1):93 (Abstr).

53. Jacquemier J, Seradour B, Hassoun J, et al. Special morphological features of invasive mammary carcinomas in women under 40 years of age. Breast Dis 1985; 1:119-122.

54. Greening WP, Montgomery ACV, Gordon AB, Gowing NFC. Quadrantic excision and axillary node dissection without radiation therapy: the long term results of a selective policy in the treatment of Stage I breas cancer. Eur J Surg Oncol 1988; 14:221-225.

55. Paterson DA, Anderson TJ, Jack WJL, et al. Pathological features predictive of local recurrence after management by conservation of invasive breast cancer: importance of noninvasive carcinoma. Radiother Oncol 1992; 25:176-180.

56. Cutler SJ, Myers MH. Clinical classification of extent of disease in cancer of the breast. J Natl Cancer Inst 1967; 39:193-207.

57. Fisher ER, Gregorio R, Redmond C, et al. Pathologic findings from the National Surgi-

cal Adjuvant Breast Project (Protocol No. 4). I. Observations concerning the multicentricity of mammary cancer. Cancer 1975; 35:247-254.

58. Fisher ER, Sass R, Fisher B, et al. Pathologic findings from the National Surgical Adjuvant Breast Project (Protocol No. 6). II. Relation of local recurrence to multi-centricity. Cancer 1986; 57:1717-1724.

59. Fisher B, Wolmark N. Conservative surgery: the American experience. Semin Oncol 1986; 13:425-433.

60. Leung S, Otmezguine Y, Calitchi E, et al. Locoregional recurrences following radical external beam irradiation and interstitial implantation for operable breast cancer - a twenty-three year experience. Radiother Oncol 1986; 5:1-10.

61. Recht A, Connolly JL, Schnitt SJ, et al. Conservative surgery and radiation therapy for early breast cancer: results, controversies, and unsolved problems. Semin Oncol 1986; 13:434-449.

62. Kurtz JM, Jacquemier J, Amalric R, et al. Breast-conserving therapy for macroscopically multiple cancers. Ann Surg 1990; 212: 38-44.

63. Lagios MD. Multicentricity of breast carcinoma demonstrated by routine correlated serial subgross and radiographic examination. Cnacer 1977; 40:1726-1734.

64. Schnitt SJ, Connolly JL, Harris JR, Hellmann S, Cohen RB. Pathologic predictors of early local recurrence in Stage I and II breast cancer treated by primary radiation therapy. Cancer 1984; 53:1049-1057.

65. Osteen RT, Connolly JL, Recht A, et al. Identification of patients at high risk for local recurrence after conservative surgery and radiation therapy for Stage I and II breast cancer. Arch Surg 1987; 122:1248-1252.

66. Recht A, Silen W, Schnitt SJ, et al. Time-course of local recurrence following conservative surgery and radiotherapy for early stage breast cancer. Int J Radiat Oncol Biol Phys 1988; 15:255-261.

67. Harris JR, Connolly JL, Schnitt SJ, et al. The use of pathologic features in selecting the extent of surgical resection necessary for breast cancer patients treated by primary radiation therapy. Ann Surg 1985; 201:164-169.

68. Recht A, Connolly JL, Schnitt SJ, et al. The effect of young age on tumor recurrence in the treated breast after conservative surgery and radiotherapy. Int J Radiat Oncol Biol Phys 1988; 14:3-10.

69. Harris JR, Connolly JL, Schnitt SJ, Cohen RB, Hellmann S. Clinical-pathologic study of early breast cancer treated by primary radiation therapy. J Clin Oncol 1983; 1:184-189.

70. Recht A, Connolly JL, Khettry U, et al. Pathologic findings on re-excision of the primary site in breast cancer patients considered for treatment by primary radiation therapy. Cancer 1987; 59:675-681.

71. Vicini FA, Eberlein TJ, Connolly JL, et al. The optimal extent of resection for patients with Stages I or II breast cancer treated with conservative surgery and radiotherapy. Ann Surg 1991; 214:200-205.

72. Zafrani B, Vielh P, Fourquet A, et al. Conservative treatment of early breast cancer: prognostic value of the ductal in situ component and other pathological variables on local control and survival. Long-term results. Eur J Cancer Clin Oncol 1989; 25:1645-1650.

73. Bloom HJG, Richardson WW. Histological grading and prognosis in breast cancer. Br J Cancer 1957; 11:359-377.

74. Moffat FL, Ketcham AS, Robinson DS, et al. Segmental mastectomy without radiotherapy for T1 and small T2 breast carcinomas. Arch Surg 1990; 125:364-369.

75. Kurtz JM, Amalric R, Brandone H, et al. Local recurrence after breast-conserving surgery and radiotherapy. Cancer 1989; 63: 1912-1917.

76. Mate TP, Carter D, Fischer DB, et al. A clinical and histopathologic analysis of the results of conservation surgery and radiation therapy in Stage I and II breast carcinoma. Cancer 1986; 58:1995-2002.

77. Clemente CG, Boracchi P, Andreola S, et al. Peritumoral lymphatic invasion in patients with node-negative mammary duct carcinoma. Cancer 1992; 69:1396-1403.

78. Hermann RE, Esselstyn EB, Crile G Jr., et al. Results of conservative operations for breast cancer. Arch Surg 1985; 120:746-75

79. Osborne MP, Ormiston N, Harmer CL, et al. Breast conservation in the treatment of early

breast cancer. A 20-year followup. Cancer 1984; 53:349-355.

80. Haffty BG, Carter D, Flynn SD, et al. Local recurrence versus new primary: clinical analysis of 82 breast relapses and potential applications for genetic fingerprinting. Int J Radiat Oncol Biol Phys 1993; 27:575-583.

81. Kurtz JM, Jacquemier J, Torhorst J, et al. Conservative therapy for breast cancers other than infiltrating ductal carcinoma. Cancer 1989; 63:1630-1635.

82. Fisher ER, Gregorio RM, Fisher B. The pathology of invasive breast cancer. A syllabus derived from the NAtional Surgical Adjuvant Breast Project (Protocol No. 4). Cancer 1975; 36:1-85.

83. Fisher ER, Fisher B. Lobular carcinoma of the breast: an overview. Ann Surg 1977; 185: 377-385.

84. Clarke DH, Martinez AA. Identification of patients who are at risk for locoregional breast cancer recurrence after conservative surgery and radiotherapy: a review article for surgeons, pathologists, adn radiation and medical oncologists. J Clin Oncol 1992; 10:474-483.

85. Kurtz JM, Spitalier J-M, Amalric R, et al. Mammary recurrences in women younger than forty. Int J Radiat Oncol Biol Phys 1988; 15:271-276.

86. Clark GM, Dressler LG, Owens MA, et al. Prediction of relapse or survival in patients with node-negative breast cancer by DNA flow cytometry. New Engl J Med 1989; 320:627-633.

87. Ciocca DR, Clark GM, Tandon AK, et al. Heat shock protein hsp70 in patients with axillary lymph node-negative breast cancer: prognostic implications. J Natl Cancer Inst 1993; 85:570-574.

88. Allred DC, Clark GM, Elledge R, et al. Association of *p53* protein expression with tumor cell proliferation rate and clinical outcome in node-negative breast cancer. J Natl Cancer Inst 1993; 85:200-206.

89. Pujol P, Maudelonde T, Daures J-P, et al. A prospective study of the prognostic value of cathepsin D levels in breast cancer cytosol. Cancer 1993; 71:2006-2012.

90. Gilbert L, Elwood LJ, Merino M, et al. A pilot study of Pi-class glutathione S-transferase expression in breast cancer: correlation with estrogen receptor expression and prognosis in node-negative breast cancer. J Clin Oncol 1993; 11:49-58.

91. Pertschuk LP, Feldman JG, Kim DS, et al. Steroid receptor immunochemistry and amplification of *c-myc* proto-oncogene. Cancer 1993; 71:162-171.

92. Marchetti A, Buttitta F, Pellegrini S, et al. *p53* mutations and histological type of invasive breast carcinoma. Cancer Res 1993; 53: 4665-4669.

93. Royds JA, Stephenson TJ, Rees RC, Shorthouse AJ, Silcocks PB. Nm23 protein expression in ductal in situ and invasive human breast carcinoma. J Natl Cancer Inst 1993; 85:727-731.

94. Seshadri R, Firgaira FA, Horsfall DJ, et al. Clinical significance of HER-2/*neu* oncogene amplification in primary breast cancer. J Clin Oncol 1993; 11:1936-1942.

95. Weidner N, Folkman J, Pozza F, et al. Tumor angiogenesis: a new significant and independent prognostic indicator in early-stage breast carcinoma. J Natl Cancer Inst 1992; 84:1875-1886.

96. Weidner N, Semple JP, Welch WR, et al. Tumor angiogenesis and metastasis - correlation in invasive breast carcinoma. New Engl J Med 1991; 324:1-8.

97. Uppsala-Örebro Breast Cancer Study Group. Sector resection with or without postoperative radiotherapy for Stage I breast cancer: a randomized trial. J Natl Cancer Inst 1990; 82:277-282.

98. Veronesi U, Luini A, Dei M, et al. Radiotherapy after breast-preserving surgery in women with localized cancer of the breast. New Engl J Med 1993; 328:1587-1591.

99. Moffat FL, Ketcham AS. Breast-conserving surgery and selective adjuvant radiation therapy for Stage I and II breast cancer. Semin Surg Oncol 1992; 8:172-176.

100. Crile G Jr. Treatment of breast cancer by local excision. Amer J Surg 1965; 109:400-403.

101. Crile G Jr. Results of conservative treatment of breast cancer at ten and 15 years. Ann Surg 1975; 181:26-30.

102. Crile G Jr., Cooperman A, Esselstyn CB, Hermann RE. Results of partial mastectomy in 173 patients followed for from five to ten years. Surg Gynecol Obstet 1980; 150: 563-566.

103. Hermann RE, Esselstyn CB Jr., Grundfest-Broniatowski S, et al. Partial mastectomy without radiation is adequate treatment for patients with Stages 0 and I carcinoma of the breast. Surg Gynecol Obstet 1993; 177: 247-253.

104. Montague ED. Conservation surgery and radiation therapy in the treatment of operable breast cancer. Cancer 1984; 53:700-704.

105. Kurtz JM, Amalric R, Brandone H, et al. Local recurrence after breast-conserving surgery and radiotherapy. Cancer 1989; 63:1912-1917.

106. Veronesi U, Banfi A, Del Vecchio M, et al. Comparison of Halsted mastectomy with quadrantectomy, axillary dissection and radiotherapy in early breast cancer: long-term results. Eur J Clin Oncol 1986; 22:1085-1089.

107. Auchincloss H. The nature of local recurrence following radical mastectomy. Cancer 1958; 11:611-619.

108. Gilliland MD, Barton RM, Copeland EM. The implications of local recurrence of breast cancer as the first site of therapeutic failure. Ann Surg 1983; 197:284-287.

109. Toonkel LM, Fix I, Jacobson LH, Wallach CB. The significance of local; recurrence of carcinoma of the breast. Int J Radiat Oncol Biol Phys 1983; 9:33-39.

110. Aberizk WJ, Silver B, Henderson IC, Cady B, Harris JR. The use of radiotherapy for treatment of isolated locoregional recurrence of breast carcinoma after mastectomy. Cancer 1986; 58:1214-1218.

111. Deutsch M, Parsons JA, Mittal BB. Radiation therapy for local-regional recurrent breast carcinoma. Int J Radiat Oncol Biol Phys 1986; 12:2061-2065.

112. Chu FCH, Lin F-J, Kim JH, Huh SH, Garmatis CJ. Locally recurrent carcinoma of the breast. Results of radiation therapy. Cancer 1976; 37:2677-2681.

113. Schwaibold F, Fowble BL, Solin LJ, Schultz DJ, Goodman RL. The results of radiation therapy for isolated local regional recurrence after mastectomy. Int J Radiat Oncol Biol Phys 1991; 21:299-310.

114. Beck TM, Hart NE, Woodard DA, Smith CE. Local or regionally recurrent carcinoma of the breast: results of therapy in 121 patients. J Clin Oncol 1983; 1:400-405.

115. Dao TL, Nemoto T. The clinical significance of skin recurrence after radical mastectomy in women with cancer of the breast. Surg Gynecol Obstet 1963; 117:447-453.

116. Donegan WL, Perez-Mesa CM, Watson FR. A biostatistical study of locally recurrent breast carcinoma. Surg Gynecol Obstet 1966; 122:529-540.

117. Stadler B, Kogelnik HD. Local control and outcome of patients irradiated for isolated chest wall recurrences of breast cancer. Radiother Oncol 1987; 8:105-111.

118. Bedwinek JM, Lee J, Fineberg B, Ocwieza M. Prognostic indicators in patients with isolated local-regional recurrence of breast cancer. Cancer 1981; 47:2232-2235.

119. Zimmerman KW, Montague ED, Fletcher GH. Frequency, anatomical distribution and management of local recurrences after definitive therapy for breat cancer. Cancer 1966; 19:67-74.

120. Fentiman IS, Matthews PN, Davison OW, Millis RR, Hayward JL. Survival following local skin recurrence after mastectomy. Br J Surg 1985; 72:14-16.

121. Halverson KJ, Perez CA, Kuske RR, et al. Isolated local-regional recurrence of breast cancer following mastectomy: radio-therapeutic management. Int J Radiat Oncol Biol Phys 1990; 19:851-858.

122. Karabali-Dalamaga S, Souhami RL, O'Higgins NJ, Soumilas A, Clark CG. Natural history and prognosis of recurrent breast cancer. Br Med J 1978; 2:730-733.

123. Greco M, Cascinelli D, Galluzzo D, et al. Locally recurrent breast cancer after 'radical' surgery. Eur J Surg Oncol 1992; 18: 209-214.

124. Mustakallio S. Treatment of breast cancer by tumor extirpation and roentgen therapy instead of radical operation. J Fac Radiol 1954; 6:23-26.

125. Peters MV. Wedge resection with or without radiation in early breast cancer. Int J Radiat Oncol Biol Phys 1977; 2:1151-1156.

126. Clark RM, Wilkinson RH, Mahoney LJ, Reid JG, MacDonald WD. Breast cancer: a 21 year experience with conservative surgery and radiation. Int J Radiat Oncol Biol Phys 1982; 8:967-975.

127. Amalric R, Santamaria F, Robert F, et al. Radiation therapy with or without primary

limited surgery for operable breast cancer: a 20-year experience at the Marseilles Cancer Institute. Cancer 1982; 49:30-34.

128. Veronesi U, Salvadori B, Luini A, et al. Conservative treatment of early breast cancer. Long-term results of 1232 cases treated with quadrantectomy, axillary dissection and radiotherapy. Ann Surg 1990; 211:250-259.

129. Veronesi U, Saccozzi R, Del Vecchio M, et al. Comparing radical mastectomy with quadrantectomy, axillary dissection and radiotherapy in patients with small cancers of the breast. New Engl J Med 1981; 305:6-11.

130. Veronesi U, Zucali R, Luini A. Local control and survival in early breast cancer: the Milan trial. Int J Radiat Oncol Biol Phys 1986; 12:717-720.

131. Veronesi U, Banfi A, Salvadori B, et al. Breast conservation is the treatment of choice in small breast cancer: long-term results of a randomized trial. Eur J Cancer Clin Oncol 1990; 26:668-670.

132. Veronesi U, Volterrani F, Luini A, et al. Quadrantectomy versus lumpectomy for small size breast cancer. Eur J Cancer 1990; 26: 671-673.

133. Haffty BG, Toth M, Flynn S, Fischer D, Carter D. Prognostic value of DNA flow cytometry in the locally recurrent, conservatively treated breast cancer patient. J Clin Oncol 1992; 10:1839-1847.

134. Stotter A, Atkinson EN, Fairston BA, et al. Survival following locoregional recurrence after breast conservation therapy for cancer. Ann Surg 1990; 212:166-172.

135. Spitalier J-M, Gambarelli JG, Brandone H, et al. Breast-conserving surgery with radiation therapy for operable mammary carcinoma: a 25-year experience. World J Surg 1986; 10:1014-1029.

136. Abner AI, Recht A, Eberlein T, et al. Prognosis following salvage mastectomy for recurrence in the breast after conservative surgery and radiation therapy for early-stage breast cancer. J Clin Oncol 1993; 11:44-48.

137. Kurtz JM, Amalric R, Brandone H, Ayme Y, Spitalier J-M. Results of salvage surgery for mammary recurrence following breast-conserving therapy. Ann Surg 1988; 207:347-351.

138. Osborne MP, Borgen PI, Wong GY, Rosen PP, McCormick B. Salvage mastectomy for local and regional recurrence after breast-conserving operation and radiation therapy. Surg Gynecol Obstet 1992; 174:189-194.

139. Cajucom CC, Tsangaris TN, Nemoto T, et al. Results of salvage mastectomy for local recurrence after breast-conserving surgery without radiation therapy. Cancer 1993; 71:1774-1779.

140. Recht A, Schnitt SJ, Connolly JL, et al. Prognosis following local or regional recurrence after conservative surgery and radiotherapy for early stage breast carcinoma. Int J Radiat Oncol Biol Phys 1989; 16:3-9.

141. Kurtz JM, Spitalier J-M, Amalric R. Late breast recurrence after lumpectomy and irradiation. Int J Radiat Oncol Biol Phys 1983; 9:1191-1194.

142. Osborne MP. Salvage mastectomy. Semin Surg Oncol 1991; 7:291-295.

143. Haffty BG, Fischer D, Beinfield M, McKhann C. Prognosis following local recurrence in the conservatively treated breast cancer patient. Int J Radiat Oncol Biol Phys 1991; 21: 293-298.

144. Stotter AT, McNeese MD, Ames FC, Oswald MJ, Ellerbroek NA. Predicting the rate and extent of locoregional failure after breast conservation therapy for early breast cancer. Cancer 1989; 64:2217-2225.

145. Chauvet B, Lemseffer A, Fetissoff F, et al. Disappearance of the in situ component: a criterion predictive of metastasis in breast cancer after local relapse. Radiother Oncol 1992; 25:181-185.

146. Kurtz JM, Amalric R, Brandone H, Ayme Y, Spitalier J-M. Results of wide excision for mammary recurrence after breast-conserving therapy. Cancer 1988; 61:1969-1972.

147. Stotter A, Kroll S, McNeese M, et al. Salvage treatment for loco-regional recurrence following breast conservation therapy for early breast cancer. Eur J Surg Oncol 1991; 17:231-236.

148. McCready DR, Fish EB, Hiraki GY, et al. Total mastectomy is not always mandatory for the treatment of recurrent breast cancer after lumpectomy alone. Can J Surg 1992; 35:485-488.

CHAPTER 4

COSMETIC OUTCOME OF BREAST CONSERVATION

Breast conservation and radical surgery are equivalent in terms of overall survival, disease-free survival and incidence of distant metastasis. As with radical or modified radical mastectomy, conservative treatment also effectively controls locoregional disease in the vast majority of patients. For breast-conserving therapy to be an acceptable alternative to mastectomy procedures, it must pass a third critical test, that of cosmetic outcome; indeed, this is the raison d'être of this therapeutic approach.

If breast conservation were not conducive to an aesthetically pleasing result, it would have no place in the management of early breast cancer. Patients would be better served by total mastectomy as current breast reconstruction techniques give good to excellent results in most cases. Breast-conserving therapy must consistently meet a high aesthetic standard to be worth the extra time and effort as compared to total or radical mastectomy.

MEASUREMENT OF COSMETIC OUTCOME

Cosmetic outcome has been measured in several ways. Most series report cosmetic or aesthetic outcome as excellent, good, fair or poor, as assessed by physician observers. While there are minor differences between series in how these categories are defined, "excellent" usually denotes minimal to no difference in appearance between the treated and untreated breasts. A good outcome is one in which there are only minor differences in terms of symmetry, contour, skin changes (hyperpigmentation or telangiectasia) and texture (minimal subcutaneous and/or parenchymal fibrosis). The cosmetic outcome is deemed fair when the treated breast has significant distortion (retraction and/or nipple deviation), volume deficit, skin changes and/or fibrosis, but the overall result is still considered aesthetically acceptable by the physician or professional making the evaluation. A poor outcome denotes an unacceptable result as evidenced by marked deformity and asymmetry, severe skin changes, or a shrunken, fibrotic, painful, unsightly breast.[1-21]

Others have devised less observer-dependent measures of the effects of breast-conserving treatment on breast symmetry, volume, contour and retraction. Veronesi et al[22] analyzed photographic images of patients' breasts by computer for breast symmetry and volume as measured by the height of the nipples, height of the inferior profiles of the breasts and distance of the nipples from the midline. Pezner et al[23] developed a breast retraction assessment (BRA) test in which the patient stands behind a vertical clear acrylic sheet which is marked off at 1-cm intervals horizontally and vertically in a grid. With the y-axis taken as the midsternal line (jugular notch to xiphoid) and the x-axis the top of the grid, x and y coordinates are taken for each nipple with the arms in three positions. BRA is calculated for each arm position as the square root of $[(x_R - x_L)^2 + (y_R - y_L)^2]$. The treated breast is thereby compared geometrically to the untreated member for retraction. While these methods minimize observer bias through the use of mathematical models, they do not take into account such aesthetically important phenomena as altered breast texture, cutaneous hyperpigmentation, telangiectasia and dysaesthetic pain syndromes.

There are important and consistent differences in how patients, their physicians and other health care professionals perceive the aesthetic outcome of breast-conserving therapy. In series in which both patients and professionals rated the cosmetic results of breast conservation, patients almost invariably gave the more favorable assessment.[7,12,16-18,24,25] Of the patients in the European Organization for Research and Treatment of Cancer (EORTC) 10801 trial, 87% rated their cosmetic outcome as good to excellent two years after treatment. At four years, 78% of patients considered their results to be good to excellent. This compares to physician ratings of good to excellent of only 79% at two years and 69% at four years.[26] Similarly, 90% of 86 patients in the breast conservation arm of the U.S. National Cancer Institute prospective randomized trial reported good to excellent aesthetic results, as compared to only 69% good to excellent outcomes as evaluated by the medical staff.[27]

Ray et al[17] found that 92% of their patients rated their conserved breast as cosmetically excellent as compared to physician observers, who rated only 82% as excellent. Of the patients studied by Borger et al,[18] 88% reported good to excellent outcome and 90% indicated they would choose this treatment option again; this compares to only 64% good to excellent ratings given by a panel of surgeons and radiotherapy personnel.

Sneeuw et al[12] found that the assessments of patients in comparing the treated with the untreated breast were similar to those of a radiation oncologist and an oncology nurse, each of whom made independent evaluations. However, there was a significantly higher level of patient satisfaction with the cosmetic result than would be implied by the comparison data. Thus, in evaluating the aesthetic quality of the conserved breast, patients take into account factors such as body image, sexuality, feelings of femininity and other subjective psychosocial considerations which a third party cannot accurately assess.[12,16] The vast majority of patients who opt for breast conservation are quite pleased with the appearance of the treated breast.

In most series, good to excellent cosmetic outcomes as measured by physicians or other health care professionals are obtained in 80% to 90% of patients (Table 4.1). There is no question that conservative management of early breast cancer is aesthetically worthwhile, and that it is the preferred treatment option in many patients for this reason.

Cosmetic outcome is time-dependent. For at least the first three years following surgery and radiation, the treated breast will continue to undergo change in many patients.[9,15,16,26] In some series, change continues over much longer periods of time. Cosmetic evaluations at an early timepoint can therefore be misleading; for accurate analysis, repeated assessments over no less than three to five years are important (vide infra).

SURGERY AND COSMESIS

EXTENT OF RESECTION

Excessive surgical resection may be a very significant factor in some poor cosmetic results.[31] In the prospective randomized trial of Veronesi et al[22] comparing quadrantectomy plus radiation to tumorectomy plus radiation, the patients treated by quadrant resection had a significantly higher incidence of breast distortion and asymmetry than those undergoing only gross tumor excision. Thus, in terms of volume of breast tissue removed at surgery, there is a trade-off between local control and cosmesis which is clearly dem-

Table 4.1. Physician-assessed cosmetic outcomes in patients undergoing breast-conserving surgery

Series	No. Patients	Surgery	XRT Dose to Breast	XRT Boost	F/U	Excellent	Good	Fair	Poor
Delouche[28]	330	Tu	50-70 Gy	10-20 Gy ext/Ir	>2 yr	38%	39%	17%	6%
Spitalier[2]	1133	Tu	50 Gy	25 Gy ext	5 yrs	68%	19%	9%	4%
					15 yrs	51%	19%	28%	2%
Amalric[29]	275	Tu or None	60 Gy	20 Gy ext	>5 yrs	— 68% —		22%	10%
Calle[4]	96	Tu*	50 Gy	15 Gy ext	5 yrs	— 60% —		38%	2%
	120	None†	50-60 Gy	20-25 Gy ext	5 yrs	— 38% —		45%	17%
Schmidt-Ullrich[6]	115	Tu	60-70 Gy	—	2 yrs	58%	33%	7%	2%
Ryoo[7]	274	Tu or SM	50 Gy	6-20 Gy ext	2-9 yrs	34%	31%	12%	13%
Blichert-Toft[1]	93	Tu	50 Gy	10-25 Gy ext	6 yrs	31%	41%	27%	1%
Olivotto[9]	593	Tu	46-50 Gy	10-27 Gy ext/Ir	3 yrs	62%	26%	9%	3%
					5 yrs	65%	25%	7%	3%
					7 yrs	54%	24%	15%	7%
Sneeuw[12]	76	Tu	54 Gy	10 Gy ext	2-11 y	15%	45%	33%	7%
Van Limbergen[10]	142	Tu	40-85 Gy	—	>3 yrs	20%	29%	29%	22%
Wazer[13]	234	Tu	50 Gy	10-20 Gy ext	>4 yrs	41%	47%	9%	3%
Recht[14]	239	Tu	50 Gy	10-20 Gy ext	5 yrs	77%	9%	9%	5%
Danoff[30]	189	Tu	46-50 Gy	15-20 Gy ext/Ir	>2 yrs	— 91% —		7%	2%
Beadle[16]	243	Tu	46-50 Gy	15-20 Gy ext/Ir	5 yrs	77%	9%	9%	5%
Ray[17]	130	Tu	45-50 Gy	15-25 Gy ext/Ir	2 yrs	— 82% —		13%	5%
Dewar[20]	592	Tu or Q	45 Gy	15 Gy ext	2 yrs	58%	38%	— 8% —	
					5 yrs	34%	54%	— 22% —	
U.S. NCI Trial[27]	86	Tu	48.6 Gy	15-20 Gy ext/Ir	67 mos	40%	29%	20%	11%

XRT   radiotherapy   F/U followup   * for primary tumors ≤ 3 cm
Tu   tumorectomy   Gy gray   † for primary tumors > 3 cm
ext   external beam boost   Ir   [192]Ir interstitial boost
Q   quadrantectomy

onstrated in this trial. This has also been observed in retrospective analyses.[5-7,9,10,13,20,23] Tumor size contributes to adverse cosmesis in part because of the more aggressive surgical resection required.[13,15,17,20]

Surgical Technique and Cosmesis

Surgical technique is very important to cosmetic outcome. Inappropriate placement of the incision, improper closure or unwarranted drainage of the segmental mastectomy wound, and incontinuous extension of the breast incision into the axilla for lymphadenectomy have all been cited as surgical errors which contribute to adverse cosmetic results.

While the aesthetic importance of careful placement of the lumpectomy incision is intuitively obvious, there are differences of opinion on which incisions are best. Clearly, the use of a centrally placed incision (i.e. circumareolar) to resect a peripheral tumor is inappropriate; the disruption of breast tissue required in such an operation predisposes to an adverse cosmetic result because of more extensive scarring and distortion over time after treatment. Moreover, obtaining clear margins would be a surgical challenge and assurance of tumor-free margins would be more problematic. In contrast to the siting of biopsy incisions in anticipation of total mastectomy, the lumpectomy incision should be placed without regard to this consideration. The NSABP[32,33] and the summary report of the American College of Radiology, the American College of Surgeons, the College of American Pathologists and the Society of Surgical Oncology[34] advocate the use of curvilinear incisions placed directly over the breast tumor itself.

There is some debate about whether incisions for tumors in the inferior half of the breast should be radially oriented[33,35] or curvilinear with the skin lines.[34] Treatment of inferiorly situated tumors by segmental mastectomy plus radiotherapy not infrequently results in a less satisfactory breast;[10] the surgeon is probably best advised to choose the incision which is optimal for the circumstances of the individual patient (i.e. her breast size and contour) and the characteristics of her tumor.

In closing the breast incision, reapproximation of the breast parenchyma is almost never indicated as this causes significant dimpling and distortion, and accentuates the asymmetry resulting from the surgical volume deficit. Rarely, in a lumpectomy performed through a radial incision for a small inferiorly situated cancer, reapproximation of the parenchyma may help to avoid unsightly distortion of the breast with downward deviation of the nipple. In patients in whom these circumstances are likely to be encountered at surgery, a radial incision is necessary as parenchymal closure through a transversely oriented incision would exacerbate the breast distortion.

In all other situations, only the subcutaneous tissues and skin of the breast should be closed, leaving the parenchymal defect to fill with fluid which subsequently undergoes organization with fibrous tissue. In this way, some of the volume deficit resulting from surgery is mitigated. Placement of a drain in the lumpectomy defect is counterproductive; evacuation of fluid from the breast defect accentuates dimpling and distortion of the residual breast tissue, and exacerbates the asymmetry of the breasts.

In general, incisions for breast resection and axillary dissection should be made separately. Extension of the lumpectomy incision into the axilla has been identified as a significant factor in adverse cosmetic outcomes.[10,32-36] However, this practice is not absolutely proscribed. In some circumstances, the axilla can be dissected through an upper outer quadrant lumpectomy incision without extension of the wound, with very favorable results. Tumors situated in the axillary tail of Spence can be resected with the axillary nodes through one incision without adverse cosmetic consequences, in the experience of this author and others.[34]

Primary Tumor Re-excision Following Diagnostic Biopsy

Re-excision of the primary tumor site following excisional biopsy has also been cited as a risk factor for adverse cosmetic outcome. Wazer et al[13] found this to be significant on univariate analysis, but patients in whom the primary site was re-excised and then a boost given to the tumor bed fared worse than those treated with either re-excision or a boost only. Re-excised patients in whom a boost was not used had better cosmetic results than those who had boosts without re-excision, although this difference did not reach statistical significance. While re-excision does result in additional sacrifice of breast volume, the data reviewed in chapter 2 on residual cancer in re-excision specimens argue for this practice, especially when histopathologically tumor-free margins of resection are sought.

Although a one-stage excision of the primary tumor has been strongly advocated,[33] not infrequently the diagnosis of infiltrating carcinoma or the discovery of a positive surgical margin is made only on examination of permanent tissue sections several days after biopsy. Routine resection of margins on the presumption of cancer for all diagnostic excisional biopsies would not be appropriate practice, as in the great majority of cases the pathology proves to be benign.[37] Careful re-excision of a biopsy or lumpectomy site is indicated when one or more margins are involved by tumor, when significant uncertainty exists in the mind of the surgeon about margin status, when the excision has been performed at another institution or when the treating surgeon is not familiar with the surgical expertise and routines of the practitioner who performed the initial biopsy procedure. A careful re-excision, even though the previous scar must be excised en bloc, should not be a major factor in cosmetic outcome in most cases.

AXILLARY LYMPHADENECTOMY AND COSMETIC RESULT IN THE BREAST

Axillary dissection is associated with a risk of ipsilateral upper extremity edema (see chapter 5) and has been identified by some as a significant factor in patients with only fair or poor cosmetic results with respect to the conserved breast. Clarke et al[38] correlated postoperative breast edema with the number of axillary nodes removed. In contrast, Wazer et al[13] found that axillary lymphadenectomy had no effect on cosmesis; in their analysis,

they took into account not only whether axillary dissection was performed, but also the volume of tissue removed from the axilla, whether there were nodal metastases on histopathology and the total number of nodes removed. Beadle et al[16] noted that limited axillary dissection, while associated with an increased likelihood of mild transient breast edema, had no effect on overall cosmesis at four years. In a subsequent report of a larger number of patients and longer followup from the same institution, Rose et al[15] confirmed that the effects of axillary lymphadenectomy on cosmesis were confined to increased early breast edema, which tended to subside with further followup. Schmidt-Ullrich et al[6] reported transient breast edema in 40% of patients during the first year after treatment, which gradually disappeared with further followup.

RADIOTHERAPY AND COSMESIS

WHOLE BREAST IRRADIATION

High radiation doses to the whole breast are prejudicial to good cosmetic results.[6,31,39] Evidence for this can be found in the cosmetic outcomes of patients treated with more than 50 Gy to the whole breast, as given in Table 4.1. Delouche et al[28] noted that the majority of patients with poor cosmesis in their series received more than 60 Gy whole breast irradiation. Of those treated with 70 Gy, 91.3% developed severe changes in the breast as compared to 33% of patients treated with 60 Gy and 11.7% of those receiving 50 Gy. Van Limbergen et al,[10] in a series in which a wide range of whole breast doses was employed, noted that those treated with whole breast irradiation to a dose of 40 to 50 Gy had uniformly excellent results, whereas none of those treated to 80 Gy had an excellent outcome and only 15% obtained a good result. Large radiation fractions (2.5 Gy to 6 Gy) were also highly deleterious to cosmesis in this series, as was the practice of preoperative "flash" radiotherapy in which five 4.0 Gy fractions of Cobalt-60 radiation were administered in one week.

RADIATION BOOST
TO THE PRIMARY TUMOR SITE

The use of a boost to the tumor bed has been identified as an adverse factor in cosmetic outcome by some authors[9,13-16,28] but was not significant in other analyses.[5,7] Olivotto et al[9] noted that cosmesis suffered progressively as the volume of tissue implanted increased, although the more extensive resections in patients with large implanted volumes were likely a confounding influence in this study. Wazer et al[13] reported that 60% of patients treated without a boost had good to excellent cosmetic results as compared to approximately 40% of patients boosted with either interstitial ^{192}Ir or electrons (p = 0.005). Patients who underwent re-excision followed by external beam elec-

Fig. 4.1 Comparison of the influence on cosmetic outcome of three-field radiotherapy (anterior regional nodal plus two tangential whole breast fields) to tangential whole breast fields only. Reproduced from Olivotto IA, et al. Int J Radiat Oncol Biol Phys 1989; 17:747-753, © 1989 with kind permission from Elsevier Science Ltd., The Boulevard, Langford Lane, Kidlington OX5 1GB, U.K.

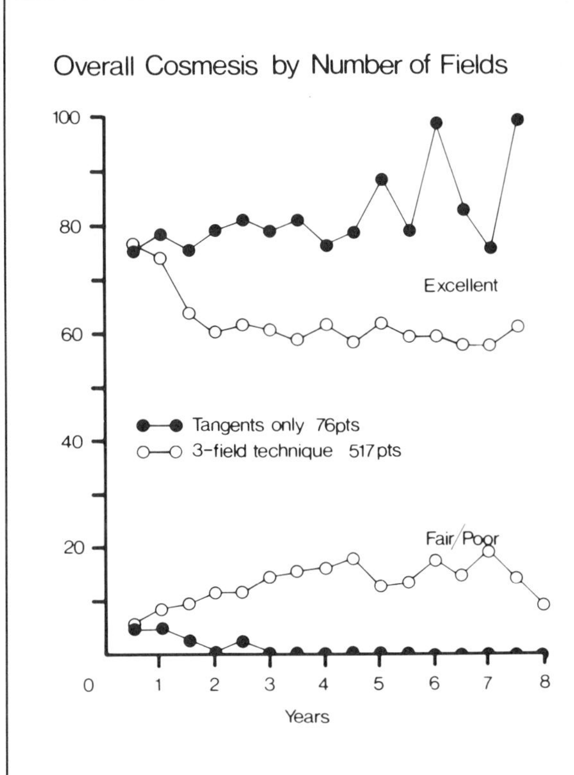

tron boost fared the worst. Beadle et al[16] noted that the use of a boost resulted in a higher incidence of telangiectasia and breast retraction at four years' followup, and that ^{192}Ir implants of larger volume (over 100 seeds) and higher dose (over 18 Gy) tended to compromise the cosmetic result.

There does not seem to be a clear consensus on whether there is any cosmetic advantage related to the choice of external beam electrons or photons as compared to brachytherapy to boost the radiation dose to the tumor bed. In the experience of some authors, cosmetic outcome with interstitial implants has not been as good as that with external beam boosts.[9,10,16,17,20,40,41] Olivotto et al[9] reported excellent cosmetic outcome at three years in 85% of patients boosted with external beam therapy as compared to only 58% of patients treated by ^{192}Ir implant (p = 0.03). A lower proportion of excellent outcomes persisted at five years, although the difference was not significant. Ray et al[17] reported a similar experience in 23 patients treated with interstitial ^{192}Ir or [226]Ra as compared to 107 patients given an external beam boost; however, the group treated with brachytherapy had larger tumors and a higher rate of grossly incomplete excisions. Six implanted patients developed functionally significant myositis of the pectoralis major muscle and six others treated for medial lesions developed radiation-related rib fractures and soft tissue problems in the volume encompassed by the boost. It should be noted that, unlike external beam irradiation, an interstitial implant results in multiple cutaneous scars at the points of insertion of the afterloading catheters. These can have a deleterious effect on the aesthetic appearance of the treated breast.

On the other hand, Delouche et al[28] concluded that interstitial ^{192}Ir was preferable to external electrons because of a higher incidence of unacceptable skin changes (i.e. telangiectasia) with the latter. Wazer et al[13] noted a trend (p = 0.09) in favor of better cosmetic outcome in patients boosted with interstitial ^{192}Ir as compared to those treated with external beam boosts, despite higher boost doses (20 Gy versus 13.7 Gy with external beam boosts, p = 0.00001) and larger tumors (33% versus 27% T2 lesions, p = 0.045) in implanted patients.

USE OF MULTIPLE RADIATION FIELDS

Irradiation of three or more fields (two tangential fields for whole breast irradiation plus one or more regional nodal fields) may have adverse cosmetic consequences because of matchline fibrosis and other effects.[7,9,10,13] Ryoo et al[7] reported that patients in whom a "hockey stick" field to treat regional lymph nodes was employed had significantly fewer good to excellent cosmetic outcomes as compared to those in whom the nodes were not irradiated. Olivotto et al[9] reported 89% excellent results at five years in patients treated only with tangential paired radiation fields

to the breast only as compared to 59% of patients in whom an additional nodal field was added (p = 0.004) (Fig. 4.1). On multivariate analysis, Van Limbergen et al[10] found that patients who received only whole breast irradiation had significantly better results than those who also had the regional nodes radiated. Patients undergoing both axillary dissection and regional nodal irradiation had the worst cosmetic outcomes by far; 62.5% had an unacceptable result, and none attained an excellent outcome. Wazer et al[13] also documented a statistically significant deleterious effect of regional nodal irradiation on long term cosmesis. Matchline fibrosis was not a prominent finding among these patients; the authors suggested that the permanent cosmetic deficits produced by overlapping radiation fields may be a function of impairment of lymphatic collateralization.

Table 4.2. The effects of postoperative adjuvant systemic chemotherapy on cosmetic outcome in patients treated by breast-conserving therapy

Series	No. Patients		Time of Evaluation	%Excellent/Good			% Fair/Poor			Comments
	no CT	CT		no CT	CT	p	no CT	CT	p	
Beadle[19]	49	49	6 mos	83*	74*	.27	—	—	—	Most of the downward
			24 mos	64*	24*	.0002	—	—	—	shift in cosmesis was
			36 mos	50*	20*	.19	22	40	.47	from excellent to good.
Rose[15]	359	134	3 yrs	68*	37*	<.0001	9	24	.004	Concurrent CT/XRT
			5 yrs	71*	40*	.001	8	20	.09	much worse than sequential CT/XRT.
Abner[44]	170	170	3 yrs	71*	47*	<.00001	9	17	.06	Concurrent CT/XRT worse than sequential. No difference between CMF and doxorubicin-based CT.
Wazer[13]	192	42	≈4 yrs	—	—	NS	—	—	NS	
Danoff[21]	19	27	≈2 yrs	89	81	.38	10	18	NS	
Hallahan[5]	166	34	3 yrs	93	91	NS	7	3	NS	CMF or CAF "sandwiched" with XRT.
Borger[18]	41	17	33 mos	—	—	NS	—	—	NS	More fibrosis in boost volume in CT patients.

* these figures are "excellent" results only; "good" not included.
CMF cyclophosphamide, methotrexate and 5-fluorouracil
NS   not statistically significant

XRT radiotherapy
CAF cyclophosphamide, doxorubicin and 5-fluorouracil
CT   chemotherapy

In contrast, Hallahan et al[5] reported no adverse cosmetic consequences in patients in whom both the breast and regional lymphatics were irradiated. However, median followup was only 36 months.

OTHER RADIOTHERAPY TECHNIQUES AND COSMESIS

Other radiotherapy-related factors which enhance cosmetic outcome include the use of anterior breast wedges to minimize dose inhomogeneities,[7] reducing tangential breast field separation (and therefore dose inhomogeneity),[13] and avoidance of radiation protocols in which tangential fields are irradiated on alternate days.[7,20]

TIME DEPENDENCE OF COSMETIC OUTCOME

Whereas most of the adverse cosmetic impact of excessive resection or suboptimal surgical technique is apparent within the first few months after treatment, the effects of radiotherapy, especially when higher dosages are used, evolve over a period of years. Fibrosis, retraction and cutaneous telangiectasia are the predominant late cosmetic effects of radiotherapy, resulting in a gradual deterioration in appearance and consistency of the breast in affected patients.[2,9,10,13,15,20,26,30] As noted above, the conserved breast continues to undergo changes for at least three years following completion of locoregional treatment.[14,16] Several series have documented ongoing changes in cosmetic outcome as late as the second decade posttreatment.[2,9,10,20,30,42,43] The magnitude of the change can be quite significant from the physician's perspective (Table 4.1), although once again it is noteworthy that even when aware of a slow deterioration in cosmesis, patients still tend to rate and value the conserved breast very highly.

Beadle et al[16] documented telangiectasia in 2% of their patients at six months followup, 33% at 30 months and 36% at 60 months. In the series of Kurtz et al,[42] 6 of 236 patients continued to show progression in breast fibrosis and/or cutaneous telangiectasia more than 10 years after treatment. Gray et al[43] noted less breast edema but more telangiectasia at five years followup. Dewar et al[20] noted a slowly progressive increase in breast asymmetry due to fibrosis over the first 10 years of followup.

ADJUVANT SYSTEMIC THERAPY AND COSMESIS

CYTOTOXIC CHEMOTHERAPY

A question has arisen over the past several years as to whether Stage II and high-risk Stage I breast cancer patients treated with postoperative adjuvant radiotherapy and chemotherapy have less satisfactory aesthetic results with breast conservation than patients receiving only radiation therapy. Straus et al,[27] in a recent report of the U.S. National Cancer Institute (NCI) trial of breast conservation versus radical surgery, noted that there was a decreased number of excellent cosmetic outcomes among patients in the breast conservation arm who also received postoperative adjuvant chemotherapy, although this did not reach statistical significance. The currently available retrospective data on possible interactions of adjuvant cytotoxic chemotherapy with radiotherapy which are detrimental to cosmesis are summarized in Table 4.2.

The three retrospective studies which report that chemotherapy is detrimental to cosmesis are all from the Joint Center for Radiation Therapy at the Harvard Medical School. The most common effect of chemotherapy on cosmetic outcome consisted of a time-dependent downgrading of cosmetic results from excellent to good; as in the NCI trial, the clinically significant effect of chemotherapy on cosmesis was modest. The preponderance of the chemotherapy effect was seen in patients treated with cytotoxic therapy and radiation concurrently rather than sequentially. Because of this and the adverse hematological consequences of concurrent therapy, sequential or "sandwich" chemotherapy-radiotherapy-chemotherapy protocols are now preferred by most radiotherapists and medical oncologists.

Of the negative studies, that of Wazer et al[13] employed CMF (cyclophosphamide, methotrexate and 5-fluorouracil) or CAF (doxorubicin instead of methotrexate) chemotherapy regimens in most patients, in which the chemotherapy was given before, during and after radiation except for the methotrexate, which was withheld during radiation therapy. Borger et al,[18] while finding no overall chemotherapy effect, documented an increase in induration of breast tissue within the tumor bed boost volume in tests of skin fold thickness.

TAMOXIFEN

Wazer et al[13] reported a marginally significant (p = 0.061) negative influence of tamoxifen on cosmetic results. Again, this was manifested primarily as a time-dependent shift in tamoxifen-treated patients from excellent to good cosmetic ratings. Among the 24 tamoxifen-treated patients in this series, the deterioration in aesthetic appearance of the breast was related to reactive fibrosis in 17, telangiectasia in five and hyperpigmentation in five. The authors speculated that a possible mechanism for this effect may relate to the fact that tamoxifen stimulates secretion of transforming growth factor β (TGFβ) in human fibroblasts. As TGFβ has been implicated in radiation-induced normal tissue fibrosis, it was proposed that tamoxifen may exacerbate the fibrotic response of normal tissues to ionizing radiations.

PATIENT FACTORS IN COSMETIC OUTCOME

THE LARGE OR FATTY BREAST

Large-breasted and obese patients are a challenge from the standpoint of cosmetic outcome.[17,43,45] Difficulties can be encountered in immobilizing a large, pendulous breast for homogeneous irradiation of the entire tissue volume in a reproducible manner over the five- to six-week treatment period. As noted above, the use of higher energy photons and wedges can assist in ensuring more uniform delivery of radiation to the breast in these individuals.

Gray et al[43] analyzed cosmetic results in "large" patients who weighed more than 80 kg, whose brassiere size was 40 inches or greater or cup size was D or larger, or in

whom the radiotherapy tangent separation was 23 cm or greater. The aesthetic outcome in 89 such patients was compared at 1, 3 and 5 years followup to that of 168 "average" women who did not meet any of the above criteria. Overall cosmesis was superior in the average group, these women demonstrating less asymmetry, fibrosis, skin thickening, retraction and late telangiectasia than the large group. While these differences were statistically significant, they were relatively small (no more than the difference between "excellent" and "good"); the authors quite appropriately concluded that large or heavy-breasted women are good candidates for breast conservation, but extra care should be taken in performing surgery and administering radiation to obtain optimal aesthetic results.

Ray et al[17] analyzed cosmetic outcome by brassiere cup size (A and B versus larger sizes) in 130 patients undergoing breast conservation treatment for early breast cancer. Of the 95 patients with small breast size, 92% had an excellent result as compared to 64% among the 45 large-breasted women. Tangent separation was a marginally significant independent variable for cosmetic result (p = 0.064).

COLLAGEN VASCULAR DISEASE

Patients with collagen vascular disease are poor candidates for breast-conserving therapy because of the high incidence of radiation-related complications and unacceptable cosmetic outcome.[46-49] These individuals are unusually prone to intense fibrotic reactions and late necrosis of irradiated bone and soft tissues.

Robertson et al[48] attempted to explain this phenomenon by postulating that the autoimmunity to type IV collagen commonly seen in these disorders may be aggravated by release of antigens from tissues exposed to ionizing radiations, probably in part through acute radiation damage to vascular endothelium. Anti-type IV collagen antibodies are mainly of the IgM class, which are potent activators of the complement system. This in turn results in an inflammatory response. Circulating monocytes migrate into the irradiated connective tissues in response to the local release of chemotactic factors, and become inflammatory macrophages. Among the cytokines secreted by these macrophages are several substances which are powerful stimulants of fibroblast proliferation and collagen synthesis, resulting in the exuberant fibrosis seen clinically.

The same process may also precipitate a worsening of the systemic manifestations of the patient's autoimmune disorder. Robertson et al[48] observed this in their breast cancer patients in concert with the progressive breast fibrosis, and suggested that antigens released by radiation gain access to the circulation through endothelial lesions within the irradiated tissue volume. The resultant autoimmune response causes a simultaneous flare-up of systemic symptoms and exacerbation of breast fibrosis.

Whatever the mechanism, it is clear that patients with a history of autoimmune reactivity or active collagen vascular disease are not amenable to adjuvant radiotherapy, and therefore for the most part should not be offered breast-conserving therapy.

REFERENCES

1. Blichert-Toft M, Rose C, Andersen JA, et al. Danish randomized trial comparing breast conservation therapy with mastectomy: six years of life-table analysis. J Natl Cancer Inst Monogr 1992; 11:19-26.
2. Spitalier JM, Gambarelli J, Brandone H, et al. Breast-conserving surgery with radiation therapy for operable mammary carcinoma: a 25 year experience. World J Surg 1986; 10:1014-1020.
3. Pierquin B, Owen R, Maylin C, et al. Radical radiation therapy of breast cancer. Int J Radiat Oncol Biol Phys 1980; 6:17-24.
4. Calle R, Pilleron JP, Schlienger P, Vilcoq JR. Conservative management of operable breast cancer. Ten years experience at the Foundation Curie. Cancer 1978; 42: 2045-2053.
5. Hallahan DE, Michel AG, Halpern HJ, et al. Breast-conserving surgery and definitive irradiation for early breast cancer. Int J Radiat Oncol Biol Phys 1989; 17: 1211-1216.
6. Schmidt-Ullrich R, Wazer D, Tercilla O, et al. Tumor margin assessment as a guide to optimal conservation surgery and irradiation in early stage breast carcinoma. Int J Radiat Oncol Biol Phys 1989; 17: 733-738.
7. Ryoo MC, Kagan AR, Wollin M, et al. Prognostic factors for recurrence and cosmesis in 393 patients after radiation therapy for early mammary carcinoma. Radiology 1989; 172:555-559.
8. Leopold KA, Recht A, Schnitt SJ, et al. Results of conservative surgery and radiation therapy for multiple synchronous cancers of one breast. Int J Radiat Oncol Biol Phys 1989; 16:11-16.
9. Olivotto IA, Rose MA, Osteen RT, et al. Late cosmetic outcome after conservative surgery and radiotherapy: analysis of causes of cosmetic failure. Int J Radiat Oncol Biol Phys 1989; 17:747-753.
10. Van Limbergen E, Rijnders A, Van der Schueren E, et al. Cosmetic evaluation of breast conserving treatment for mammary cancer. 2. A quantitative analysis of the influence of radiation dose, fractionation schedules and surgical treatment techniques on cosmetic results. Radiother Oncol 1989; 16:253-267.
11. Levitt SH. Primary treatment of early breast cancer with conservation surgery and radiation therapy. Cancer 1985; 55:2140-2148.
12. Sneeuw KCA, Aaronson NK, Yarnold JR, et al. Cosmetic and functional outcomes of breast conserving treatment for early stage breast cancer. 1. Comparison of patients' ratings, observers' ratings and objective assessments. Radiother Oncol 1992; 25: 153-159.
13. Wazer DE, DiPetrillo T, Schmidt-Ullrich R, et al. Factors influencing cosmetic outcome and complication risk after conservative surgery and radiotherapy for early-stage breast carcinoma. J Clin Oncol 1992; 10:356-363.
14. Recht A, Connolly JL, Schnitt SJ, et al. Conservative surgery and radiation therapy for early breast cancer: results, controversies and unsolved problems. Semin Oncol 1986; 13:434-449.

15. Rose MA, Olivotto I, Cady B, et al. Conservative surgery and radiation therapy for early breast cancer. Long-term cosmetic results. Arch Surg 1989; 124:153-157.

16. Beadle GF, Silver B, Botnick L, Hellman S, Harris JR. Cosmetic results following primary radiation therapy for early breast cancer. Cancer 1984; 54:2911-2918.

17. Ray GR, Fish VJ. Biopsy and definitive radiation therapy in Stage I and II adenocarcinoma of the female breast: analysis of cosmesis and the role of electron beam supplementation. Int J Radiat Oncol Biol Phys 1983; 9:813-818.

18. Borger JH, Keijser AH. Conservative breast cancer treatment: analysis of cosmetic results and the role of concomitant adjuvant chemotherapy. Int J Radiat Oncol Biol Phys 1987; 13:1173-1177.

19. Beadle GF, Come S, Henderson IC, et al. The effect of adjuvant chemotherapy on the cosmetic results after primary radiation treatment for early stage breast cancer. Int J Radiat Oncol Biol Phys 1984; 10: 2131-2137.

20. Dewar JA, Benhamou S, Benhamou E, et al. Cosmetic results following lumpectomy, axillary dissection and radiotherapy for small breast cancers. Radiother Oncol 1988; 12:273-280.

21. Danoff BF, Goodman RL, Glick JH, Haller DG, Pajak TF. The effect of adjuvant chemotherapy on cosmesis and complications in patients with breast cancer treated by definitive irradiation. Int J Radiat Oncol Biol Phys 1983; 9:1625-1630.

22. Veronesi U, Volterrani F, Luini A, et al. Quadrantectomy versus lumpectomy for small size breast cancer. Eur J Cancer 1990; 26:671-673.

23. Pezner RD, Patterson MP, Hill LR, et al. Breast retraction assessment: an objective evaluation of cosmetic results of patients treated conservatively for breast cancer. Int J Radiat Oncol Biol Phys 1985; 11: 575-578.

24. Blichert-Toft M, Brincker H, Andersen JA, et al. A Danish randomized trial comparing breast-preserving therapy with mastectomy in mammary carcinoma. Acta Oncol 1988; 27:671-677.

25. Anscher MS, Jones P, Prosnitz LR, et al. Local failure and margin status in early-stage breast carcinoma treated with conservation surgery and radiation therapy. Ann Surg 1993; 218:22-28.

26. van Dongen JA, Bartelink H, Fentiman IS, et al. Randomized clinical trial to assess the valu of breast-conserving therapy in Stage I and II breast cancer, EORTC 10801. Monogr J Natl Cancer Inst 1992; 11:15-18.

27. Straus K, Lichter A, Lippman M, et al. Results of the National Cancer Institute Early Breast Cancer Trial. Monogr J Natl Cancer Inst 1992; 11:27-32.

28. Delouche G, Bachelot F, Premont MD, Kurtz JM. Conservation treatment of early breast cancer: long term results and complications. Int J Radiat Oncol Biol Phys 1987; 13:29-34.

29. Amalric R, Santamaria F, Robert F, et al. Radiation therapy with or without primary limited surgery for operable breast cancer: a 20-year experience at the Marseilles Cancer Institute. Cancer 1982; 49:30-34.

30. Danoff BF, Pajak TF, Solin LJ, Goodman RL. Excisional biopsy, axillary node dissection and definitive radiotherapy for Stages I and II breast cancer. Int J Radiat Oncol Biol Phys 1985; 11:479-483.

31. Marcial VA. Primary therapy for limited breast cancer. Cancer 1990; 65:2159-2164.

32. Fisher B, Wolmark N, Fisher ER, Deutsch M. Lumpectomy and axillary dissection for breast cancer: surgical, pathological, and radiation considerations. World J Surg 1985; 9:692-698.

33. Fisher B. Reappraisal of breast biopsy prompted by the use of lumpectomy. J Amer Med Assoc 1985; 253:3585-3588.

34. Winchester PD, Cox JD. Standards for breast-conservation treatment. CA - A Cancer Journal for Clinicians 1992; 42:134-162.

35. Harris JR, Hellman S, Kinne DW. Limited surgery and radiotherapy for early breast cancer. New Engl J Med 1985; 313: 1365-1368.

36. Smith TJ, Wazer DE, Robert NJ, Homer MJ, Safaii H. Local/regional therapy of primary breast cancer: a contemporary multimodal approach. Semin Oncol 1992; 19:230-238.

37. Moffat FL, Ketcham AS. Has mammography led to too many breast biopsies? J Surg Oncol 1990; 45:1-3.

38. Clarke D, Martinez A, Coe RS, Goffinet DR. Breast edema following staging axillary dissection in patients with breast carcinoma treated by radical radiotherapy. Cancer 1982; 49:2295-2299.

39. Fowble B. Radiotherapeutic considerations in the treatment of primary breast cancer. J Natl Cancer Inst Monogr 1992; 11:49-58.

40. Bedwinek J. Adjuvant irradiation for early breast cancer. An ongoing controversy. Cancer 1984; 53:729-739.

41. Fowble B, Solin LJ, Martz KL, et al. The influence of the type of boost (electrons vs. implant) on local control and cosmesis in patients with stages I and II breast cancer undergoing conservative surgery and radiation. Int J Radiat Oncol Biol Phys 1986; 12:150.

42. Kurtz JM, Amalric R, Delouche, et al. The second ten years: long-term risks of breast conservation in early breast cancer. Int J Radiat Oncol Biol Phys 1987; 13: 1327-1332.

43. Gray JR, McCormick B, Cox L, Yahalom J. Primary breast irradiation in large-breasted of heavy women: analysis of cosmetic outcome. Int J Radiat Oncol Biol Phys 1991; 21:347-354.

44. Abner AL, Recht A, Vicini FA, et al. Cosmetic results after surgery, chemotherapy and radiation therapy for early breast cancer. Int J Radiat Oncol Biol Phys 1991; 21:331-338.

45. Clarke D, Martinez A, Cox RS. Analysis of cosmetic results and complications in patients with Stage I and II breast cancer treated by biopsy and irradiation. Int J Radiat Oncol Biol Phys 1983; 9:1807-1813.

46. Fleck R, McNeese MD, Ellerbroek NA, et al. Consequences of breast irradiation in patients with preexisting collagen vascular diseases. Int J Radiat Oncol Biol Phys 1989; 17:829-833.

47. Matthews RH. Collagen vascular disease and irradiation. Int J Radiat Oncol Biol Phys 1989; 17:1123-1124.

48. Robertson JM, Clarke DH, Pevzner MM, Matter RC. Breast Conservation Therapy. Severe fibrosis after radiation therapy in patients with collagen vascular disease. Cancer 1991; 68:502-508.

49. Ransom DT, Cameron FG. Scleroderma: a possible contra-indication to lumpectomy and radiotherapy in breast carcinoma. Australas Radiol 1987; 31:317-318.

CHAPTER 5

MANAGEMENT OF THE AXILLARY LYMPHATICS IN EARLY INVASIVE BREAST CANCER

Axillary lymph node status is the most significant pathological determinant of prognosis in patients with early stage breast cancer.[1-3] Patients with axillary nodal metastases are much more likely to develop systemic metastases and die of their disease than those with no nodal involvement. More than any other single factor, the discovery that postoperative systemic adjuvant therapy significantly reduces the risk of breast cancer dissemination and death in node-positive patients[4-8] has made histopathological evaluation of the axillary lymph nodes imperative. Even patients with infiltrating carcinomas of 5 mm or less in size have approximately a one-in-five chance of harboring metastatic tumor in the ipsilateral axilla, which puts them at much higher risk for breast cancer relapse and mortality than node-negative patients with infiltrating carcinomas of similar size (see Table 7.1).

The experience of the National Surgical Adjuvant Breast Project (NSABP) clearly demonstrates that, although there is a significant increment in incidence of subsequent distant metastasis and disease-specific mortality between patients with three or fewer positive nodes and those with four or more,[2] these hazards behave as continuous variables. The incidence of tumor dissemination and breast cancer deaths rises steadily as the total number of involved axillary lymph nodes increases.[3] The most recent clinicopathological analyses of the NSABP B-04 and B-06 studies confirm these earlier observations. Ten-year survival of patients in the B-04 trial with 0, 1 to 3, 4 to 9, and 10 or more involved axillary nodes was 67%, 47%, 30% and 12%.[9] For B-06 node-positive patients these figures were 75%, 62%, 42% and 20%, respectively.[10] It must be remembered that node-positive patients in the B-04 trial received no adjuvant systemic therapy (the time period over which patients were entered into this trial antedated demonstration of the efficacy of adjuvant cytotoxic treatment). B-06 patients were treated with a now-outdated regimen of melphalan and 5-fluorouracil.

The total number of involved axillary lymph nodes has taken on additional clinical relevance with the advent of high-dose chemotherapy regimens and autologous stem cell support or bone marrow transplantation.[11] Patients with 10 or more involved nodes have a 60% to 90% ten-year risk of treatment failure with current conventional adjuvant chemotherapy; these individuals are therefore considered candidates for these radical protocols.[3,12,13] Early experience with high-dose chemotherapy and autologous stem cell support has provided grounds for hope that radical systemic treatment may significantly improve the prospects for cure in these high-risk patients.[14,15] However, at present such therapy carries a significant risk of major morbidity and even mortality; it is important that only patients with a large number of nodal metastases be accepted into such protocols.

Fisher et al,[16] in an analysis of nodal staging and extent of axillary surgery using data from the NSABP B-04 trial, showed that as the total number of nodes resected from the axilla increases, the proportion of pathological node-positive patients with four or more involved nodes also rises. The surgical procedure used to stage the axilla should therefore be of sufficient magnitude to yield a generous number of lymph nodes for histopathological examination; only then can triage of individual patients for appropriate adjuvant systemic therapy proceed with confidence.

Several prospective randomized trials[17-20] have demonstrated that some subsets of node-negative breast cancer patients may also benefit from postoperative adjuvant cytotoxic chemotherapy or tamoxifen. Chemotherapy protocols for Stage I breast cancer tend to be less intensive, of shorter duration,[20] and may not include alkylating agents such as cyclophosphamide[17] which are routinely included in adjuvant therapy for pathological node-positive disease. Such regimens are acceptable for use in Stage I breast cancer patients in part because of the reduced incidence and severity of morbidity associated with them. Therefore, contrary to the expectations of some, the advent of adjuvant cytotoxic therapy for node-negative disease has not relieved oncologists of the obligation to determine pathological axillary nodal status prior to making recommendations regarding adjuvant systemic therapy.

Clinical evaluation of the axilla for the presence or absence of metastatic breast cancer is inherently inaccurate, especially when the axillary lymph nodes are clinically benign or nonpalpable (Table 5.1). Chevinsky et al[27] found that clinical assessment of the axillary lymphatics for the presence of metastases had a sensitivity of only 42%. Kitchen et al[28] reported that of 100 consecutive pathological node-positive breast cancer patients, preoperative clinical evaluation correctly identified the presence of axillary metastases in only 38. Fisher et al[16] reported

Table 5.1. Inaccuracy of clinical evaluation of the axillary lymphatics for metastatic involvement by breast cancer

Series	No. Patients	Pathological Error Associated with Clinical Nodal Status	
		Clinical False-Negative*	Clinical False-Positive†
NSABP B-04[16]	641	38.6%	27.3%
Danforth[21]	136	37.6%	11.1%
Ball[22]	237	45%	20%
Lin[23]	283	28%	14%
Rose[24]	176	22%	9%
Cutler[25]	1210‡	41.6%	27%
	1917§	38.4%	32.7%
Davies[26]	149	34%	33%

* Incidence of pathological node-positive patients among those judged to be node-negative on clinical examination.

† Incidence of pathological node-negative patients among those judged to be node-positive on clinical examination.

‡ Patients operated upon at Memorial Hospital, New York.

§ Patients from the Surveillance, Epidemiology and End Results group.

that of the clinical node-negative patients in the NSABP B-04 trial who proved to be pathologically node-positive, almost one-half had four or more involved nodes. Axillary nodal status can be precisely determined only by surgical removal and histopathological evaluation of the ipsilateral axillary lymphatics.

It is also of considerable importance that axillary disease be effectively controlled and recurrence in the axilla thereby prevented. While infrequent in most series, axillary relapse can be difficult to detect in the presence of posttreatment changes in the axilla. Unfortunately, recurrent axillary breast cancer may not be discovered until the major neurovascular structures to the ipsilateral upper extremity have been encroached upon or invaded by tumor.[29-31] The risk of axillary relapse may be particularly high in patients with palpable axillary metastases or gross evidence of nodal involvement[32,33] at the time of axillary lymphadenectomy. It is noteworthy that, while occult or micrometastatic involvement of the axillary nodes may have only a small adverse effect on survival, treatment failure is much more common in pathological node-positive than node-negative patients irrespective of whether the axillary disease is microscopic or gross.[32-36]

It is unclear whether extranodal extension of tumor is an independent risk factor for axillary relapse in breast cancer patients.[37,38] However, extracapsular invasion is associated with extensive, macroscopic axillary disease which, as noted above, connotes a high risk for axillary relapse.

Management of the axilla in patients with early breast cancer is an ongoing focus of controversy. Rapid advances in adjuvant systemic therapy such as those discussed above have only re-energized the debate over what constitutes the optimal therapeutic approach to the axillary lymphatics. Management options employed in the past have included axillary node biopsy or sampling,[26,39-45] partial axillary lymphadenectomy,[45-50] total axillary lymphadenectomy,[29,51-59] and radiotherapy used alone or in combination with surgery.[48,51,59-63]

There has been a recent spate of reports in favor of limited axillary intervention based on observation of effective control of axillary disease (especially when limited surgery is used in combination with radiotherapy),[45,48,49,62] accurate disease staging using only axillary sampling procedures,[39,40-42] and reduced long term morbidity.[49] Proponents of conservative axillary treatment are quick to point out that their approach is consistent in spirit with breast conservation therapy for primary breast cancer.

Treatment of the axillary lymphatics is addressed here in light of these new developments in adjuvant systemic therapy, the consequent increased importance of precise quantitative nodal staging, disease control in the axilla and the morbidity of the various therapeutic approaches to the axillary nodes.

THE AXILLARY LYMPHATICS

The relevant surgical anatomy of the axilla is shown in Figure 5.1. Berg[64] divided the axilla into three levels for purposes of surgical identification and prognostication. Whether level of nodal involvement is an independent predictor of prognosis has been disputed, and now appears doubtful. Nonetheless, Berg's levels, designated I, II and III and defined by the medial and lateral borders of the pectoralis minor muscle, are useful as points of reference in discussing axillary lymphadenectomy for breast cancer.

Level I nodes are those found lateral to the lateral border of the muscle and inferior to the axillary vein in the fat pad which occupies the space anterior to the subscapularis and latissimus dorsi muscles. The intercostobrachial nerves, which are sensory to the axillary skin and the medial aspect of the proximal upper extremity, traverse this fat pad. They are either sacrificed in the course of resecting these nodes or, in the absence of gross evidence of metastatic tumor, can be dissected out and spared.[65]

Level II nodes are found behind the pectoralis minor muscle. While their position is anatomically clear, the delineation of these nodes is very nebulous from the surgeon's point of view. The retraction of one or both pectoral muscles which is necessary to perform the operation makes distinc-

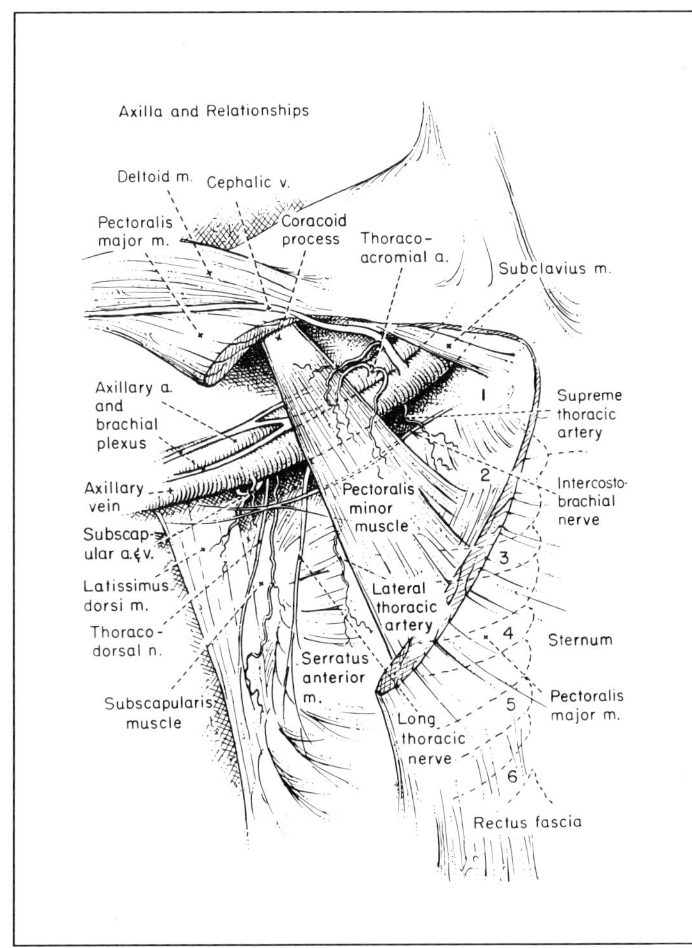

Fig. 5.1. The surgical anatomy of the axilla. The pectoralis major muscle is cut away, exposing the underlying pectoralis minor muscle, the lateral and medial borders of which divide the axillary lymphatics into Berg's levels I, II and III. The subclavius muscle invested by the clavipectoral fascia, referred to in the surgical literature as Halsted's ligament, extends from the first rib to the undersurface of the clavicle. This structure represents the upper limit of dissection for a total (levels I, II and III) axillary lymphadenectomy. The long thoracic and thoracodorsal nerves are routinely preserved unless directly involved by metastatic cancer. Some surgeons preserve the intercostobrachial neuro-vascular bundles when there is little or no gross disease in the axilla. Reproduced with permission from Southwick HW, Slaughter DP, Humphrey LJ. Surgery of the Breast. Year Book Medical Publishers (Mosby-Year Book, Inc.), Chicago, 1968. p 21.

tion of level I from level II nodes a highly arbitrary exercise. Many surgeons who prefer lymphadenectomy to node sampling procedures resect level I and II nodes en bloc.

The apical or level III nodes reside medial to the pectoralis minor and inferior to the axillary vein, and extend medially and superiorly to Halsted's ligament (the subclavius muscle invested by the clavipectoral fascia). But for the presence of Halsted's ligament, these nodes would be continuous with the supraclavicular nodes. The level III lymph nodes can be exposed for resection by either retracting the pectoral muscles anteriorly or by dividing the coracoid insertion of pectoralis minor; the latter maneuver is of little or no functional consequence. If there is massive disease throughout the axillary lymphatics, the level III nodes and pectoralis minor are best resected en bloc with levels I and II. In these circumstances, care must be taken not to injure or divide the lateral pectoral neurovascular bundle as it crosses the lateral border of pectoralis minor; the resultant atrophy of pectoralis major can contribute to an adverse cosmetic and/or functional result.[66]

The interpectoral or Rotter's nodes, routinely resected with the pectoral muscles in the Halsted radical mastectomy, are found along the medial pectoral neurovascular bundle. These are accessible to resection during axillary dissection in breast conserving operations by simply opening the interpectoral groove and carefully dissecting out the fat pad which lies along the medial pectoral vessels. Resection of Rotter's lymph nodes is performed routinely by some surgeons, adds almost no time to the procedure and has little or no associated morbidity.[51,52,67,68]

The number of lymph nodes obtained in axillary staging procedures varies greatly, ranging from as few as five to as many as 60 lymph nodes when a total axillary lymphadenectomy (levels I, II and III with or without interpectoral nodes) has been performed.[21,27,51] This wide range is a function of biological variability in the number of nodes in individual patients, the extent of surgical resection (sampling versus partial or total axillary dissection), the thoroughness with which the surgeon clears the lymphatic tissue from the region(s) of the axilla being dissected, and the diligence of the pathologist in searching for and identifying lymph nodes in the submitted tissues. Therefore, published data on the number of lymph nodes removed from the axilla is of limited value in determining the extent of the axillary staging procedure employed.

Detailed descriptions of surgical procedures and the methods by which nodes are examined by the pathologist are of far greater value when comparing results between series. Precise disclosure of the anatomical boundaries of resection eliminates ambiguity about the extent of surgery irrespective of the number of nodes identified.

SENSITIVITY OF AXILLARY STAGING PROCEDURES

Table 5.2 summarizes currently available information on the distribution of metastatic disease in the axillary lymphatics of node-positive breast cancer patients undergoing total axillary lymphadenectomy as defined above. In the majority of patients, spread of tumor into the axilla proceeds in an orderly fashion, progressively moving into higher lymph node levels as metastatic involvement becomes more extensive.[29,30,32] However, in 0.1% to 5.5% of pathological node-positive patients (9.9% and 11.4% in two series[55,56]), the apical and/or Rotter's lymph nodes are the only sites of metastatic disease in the axilla.

AXILLARY BIOPSY AND SAMPLING

Axillary sampling procedures have been promoted as operations which for purposes of nodal staging provide information equivalent

---

Table 5.2. Incidence of apical (level III) and Rotter's (interpectoral) nodal metastases in pathological node-positive (pN+) breast cancer patients

Series	No. of Axillae	No. of pN+ Axillae	No. with Apical Metastases	No. with Rotter's Metastases	No. with "Skip" Metastases*
Danforth[21]	136	65	18 (27.7%)	— —	2 (3.1%)
Chevinsky[27]	204	93	36 (38.7%)	— —	2 (2.2%)
Veronesi[29]	—	539	102 (18.9%)	— —	2 (0.4%)
Veronesi[30]	1446	839	186 (22.2%)	— —	1 (0.1%)
Senofsky[51]	278	92	24 (26.1%)	14 (15.2%)	5 (5.5%)
Rosen[52]	1228	429	104 (24.2%)	1 (0.2%)	15 (3.5%)
Schwartz[53]	277	127	— —	— —	4 (3.1%)
Pigott[54]	146	72[†]	30 (41.7%)	— —	3 (4.1%)
Attiyeh[55]	—	105	61 (58.1%)	— —	12 (11.4%)
Smith[56]	408	304	136 (44.7%)	— —	30 (9.9%)
Boova[58]	200	80	17 (21.2%)	— —	1 (1.2%)
Cody[67]	500	134	— —	13 (9.7%)	— —
Gaglia[69]	492	255	75 (29.4%)	— —	6 (2.4%)
Toma[70]	185	108	31 (28.7%)	— —	0 (0%)
Barth[71]	135	64	17 (26.5%)	— —	2 (3.1%)

Percentages in parentheses pertain to pN+ patients.
* "Skip" metastases are defined as tumor in apical (level III) and/or Rotter's nodes in the absence of metastatic involvement of level I and II lymph nodes.
† 72 evaluable patients of a total of 80 pN+ patients in this series.
Adapted from Moffat FL, et al. J Surg Oncol 1992; 51:8-13 © 1992, Wiley-Liss

to that obtained by partial axillary lymphadenectomy or total axillary lymphadenectomy. Most of these operations sample the lower axillary nodes either randomly or as directed by palpation of the axillary contents at the time of surgery. Steele et al[39] compared axillary sampling to "axillary clearance" in a prospective randomized trial. Axillary sampling involved careful definition and dissection of the axillary tail of the breast and immediately adjacent axillary tissues. Sampling procedures yielded a mean of 5 nodes as compared to 21 nodes with clearance. In the last 135 patients, randomization to sampling only or full clearance was carried out intraoperatively after mastectomy and sampling had been completed. The proportion of patients identified as pathological node-positive was reported to be virtually identical in each group.

However, Cant et al,[42] in sampling the axillary tail of the breast and lower axilla by a similar technique, failed to identify any lymph nodes in resected axillary tissue in 10% of patients in their series. Forrest et al[43] were unable to identify lymph nodes in sampled axillary tissue in 13% of studied patients.

In two prospective studies, sampling was found to be markedly inferior to formal axillary lymphadenectomy for nodal staging. Kissin et al[44] studied 50 consecutive patients in whom total mastectomy and sampling were first performed, and then total axillary lymphadenectomy was completed under the same anaesthetic. Sampling yielded a mean of 4 nodes (range 0 to 6) and lymphadenectomy 14 additional nodes (6 to 26) for examination. No lymph nodes were recovered in sampled axillary tissue in five patients (10%), two of whom proved to be pathological node-positive. The overall staging error with sampling was 24%, and in at least three cases the number of involved nodes was badly underestimated.

Davies et al[26] performed axillary node biopsy (one node) followed by completion axillary lymphadenectomy (24 nodes) in 54 patients, and axillary node sampling by the Forrest technique[43] (six nodes on average) followed by completion lymphadenectomy.

Biopsy reduced the clinical false-positive staging error from 33% to 19%, but failed to identify the presence of axillary metastases in 11 of 26 (42%) pathological node-positive patients. Axillary sampling failed to detect metastatic tumor in 6 of 43 (14%) pathological node-positive patients. In three of these patients, nodal involvement was limited to the higher levels of the axilla.

Thus, axillary node biopsy or sampling procedures are clearly inferior to lymphadenectomy for breast cancer staging. Moreover, given the current need for precise quantitative information on axillary nodal involvement for appropriate adjuvant systemic therapy, these procedures are wholly inadequate and should be abandoned.

PARTIAL AND TOTAL AXILLARY LYMPHADENECTOMY

A number of studies have concluded that a partial axillary lymphadenectomy (PAL) incorporating both level I and II lymph nodes provides highly reliable staging information, resulting in surgical understaging in only 0.2% to 3.1% of patients.[49,51-54,56,58,68] Resection of level I lymph nodes alone, on the other hand, would permit examination of only about half of the axillary lymph nodes. Danforth et al[21] noted that, in their 136 total axillary lymphadenectomies (TAL), 39% of examined nodes were found in level I, 41% in level II and 20% in level III. In the series of Veronesi et al, 65% of nodes were recovered from level I, 25% from level II and 10% from level III. Chevinsky et al[27] found 46% of lymph nodes in level I, 33% in level II and 21% in level III. The variations between these series can probably be attributed in large measure to the difficulty inherent in precisely distinguishing level II from levels I and III intraoperatively. In any event, it is clear that additional resection of level II nodes in PAL would greatly increase the number of lymph nodes available for examination, with a commensurate improvement in the precision of nodal staging.

In twelve series, TAL was performed and nodes were separated into the three Berg's levels. It is therefore possible from these data to compare the understaging errors of level

I versus level I and II PAL (Table 5.3). In most of these series, addition of level II to level I nodal information increases the staging sensitivity of PAL significantly; in fact, in all but one series[56] very few pathological node-positive axillae would have been missed had a partial axillary resection included both level I and II lymph nodes.

Axelsson et al[73] found that among 7,145 patients in Danish Breast Cancer Cooperative Study Group trials, the proportion of patients discovered to be pathological node-positive increased with the number of lymph nodes resected in axillary staging procedures. This direct relationship between number of nodes resected and proportion of node-positivity held up to 10 lymph nodes; the proportion of node-positive patients leveled off with larger numbers of nodes.

In series from two institutions,[29,30,52] level I PAL would have revealed the presence of axillary metastases in over 96% of node-positive patients. The discrepancy in sensitivity of level I PAL between these series and the others in Table 5.3 may be related to variations in identification and separation of level I from level II nodes.

That determination of the status of level I nodes, which includes less than 50% of the axillary nodes, should detect 70% to 96% of pathological node-positive axillae supports the general concept of progressive, stepwise

invasion of the axillary lymphatics by breast cancer.[29,30] From the standpoint of breast cancer staging, "skip" metastases are a relatively minor problem as shown in Table 5.2. The information in Table 5.3 confirms that PAL encompassing nodes from both levels I and II is more sensitive than level I PAL as a surgical staging procedure, and results in understaging in no more than 3% to 3.5% of patients. TAL of course has the highest sensitivity; removal of all axillary lymphatic tissue eliminates the surgical staging error altogether.

PREVENTION OF BREAST CANCER RELAPSE IN THE AXILLA

Axillary failures are fortunately uncommon. Such recurrences, especially those which develop in the apex of the axilla (i.e. medial to pectoralis minor) often only come to light late in their course. These present the clinician and patient with formidable, even intractable problems as they frequently involve the axillary vessels and the brachial plexus.[29-31]

The NSABP B-04 trial established that untreated, nonpalpable axillary nodal metastases do not invariably develop into regional recurrences in the course of post-treatment surveillance. However, it was also clearly demonstrated that the incidence of axillary failure in clinical node-negative patients is unacceptably high when the axilla

Table 5.3. Proportion of pathological node-positive (pN+) patients which would escape detection by level I as compared to level I and II partial axillary lymphadenectomy

		Understaging Error by Partial Axillary Lymphadenectomy (PAL)	
Series	**No. pN+ Axillae**	**Level I PAL**	**Level I and II PAL**
Danforth[21]	136	29.2%	3.1%
Chevinsky[27]	93	8.6%	2.2%
Veronesi[29]	539	1.5%	0.4%
Veronesi[30]	839	1.3%	0.1%
Rosen[52]	429	3.9%	1.8%
Schwartz[53]	127	13.4%	3.2%
Pigott[54]	72	25.0%	1.4%
Smith[56]	408	29.0%	13.0%
Boova[58]	80	8.8%	1.2%
Gaglia[69]	255	15.0%	2.5%
Toma[70]	108	10.2%	0%
Barth[71]	64	29.7%	3.1%

is not treated at all. Of the clinical node-negative patients in the radical mastectomy arm of the B-04 study, 39% were found to have one or more histopathologically involved axillary nodes. This compares to 18% of clinical node-negative patients treated by total mastectomy without axillary intervention who went on to develop clinical axillary relapse in the course of followup.[47,50] Oncologists of all disciplines would agree that axillary intervention to abrogate a 20% risk of regional nodal relapse in clinical node-negative breast cancer patients is worthwhile.

As already noted, treatment failure including axillary relapse is more likely when the axillary nodes are microscopically or grossly invaded by breast cancer.[32-36] Gross metastases are associated with the highest risk of axillary recurrence.[32,33] However, the absence of histopathological evidence of metastatic disease in axillary nodes removed in less-than-total axillary lymphadenectomies provides no guarantee against nodal failure. The risk of axillary relapse in pathological node-negative patients ranges from about 3% when 10 or more nodes have been resected by PAL to at least 10% when only one or two lymph nodes have been removed.[46,74]

The risk of axillary relapse is also dependent on axillary treatment (Table 5.4). Axillary radiotherapy alone effectively controls the axilla in clinical node-negative patients. However, in patients so treated no information is obtained on pathological nodal stage; these individuals may therefore not get the systemic adjuvant therapy which would be optimal for their disease. Lymphadenectomy effectively prevents axillary recurrence while providing detailed and accurate information on the histopathological status of the axillary lymphatics.

TAL probably provides better control of axillary disease than PAL; the slightly higher axillary recurrence rates in the two British trials[40,63] in which TAL was used are probably due to inclusion of patients with locoregionally advanced (Stage III) disease in these studies. Properly performed, TAL assures complete clearance of tumor from the axilla. When level III nodes are not resected, 19% to 58% of pathological node-positive patients will be left with residual disease in the axilla, as suggested by the data shown in Table 5.2. PAL with postoperative adjuvant radiotherapy is also very effective in preventing axillary recurrence, but the incidence of complications is much higher than with either surgery or radiotherapy alone (vide infra).

The NSABP B-04 trial,[16,47,50] the Danish Breast Cancer Cooperative Study Group,[46,73,74] the University of Pennsylvania/ Fox Chase Cancer Center[80] and the Joint Center for Radiation Therapy at Harvard[77] have all clearly demonstrated that the risk of cancer recurrence in the axilla is inversely related to the number of axillary lymph nodes resected. Observation only and nodal biopsy or sampling, with reported axillary nodal failure rates of 5% to 21%, are clearly inadequate for regional disease control and much inferior to PAL, TAL or axillary irradiation in this regard.[45-47,50,61] The incidence of axillary relapse after node sampling or PAL is reduced by the addition of postoperative adjuvant regional radiotherapy, albeit at the price of significantly increased long-term morbidity.[62] In the NSABP B-04 trial, axillary relapse in clinical node-positive patients treated by radical mastectomy was 1%, significantly lower than the 12% incidence observed in clinical node-positive patients treated by total mastectomy plus axillary radiotherapy (i.e. no axillary surgery).[47,50]

Patients in whom PAL is performed have at most a 2% to 4% risk of subsequent axillary failure.[45,46,48,61,62] Axillary failure following TAL is usually very rare. None of the patients in the University of Miami series has suffered an axillary relapse.[51,68] Of patients treated by TAL in a study from the Royal Marsden Hospital, none recurred in the axilla whereas the failure rate among those treated by more conservative operations or by axillary irradiation was 14.5%.[61] As already noted, only 1% of clinical node-positive patients treated by radical mastectomy in the NSABP B-04 trial had relapsed in the axilla at 10 years followup.[47,50] Kissin et al[44] reported a 1% incidence of axillary recurrence with TAL in 300 consecutive cases. Veronesi et al[29,31,57] at the Milan National Cancer Institute also reported axillary

Table 5.4. The incidence of axillary recurrence following axillary surgery and/or radiotherapy

Axillary Intervention	No. Patients	Nodal Stratification	Followup	Axillary Recurrence
Observation Only				
Graversen[46]	193	—	6.5 yrs	19%
NSABP B-04[47]	365	cN–	10 yrs	18%
Axillary Biopsy/Sampling				
Forrest[40]	75	—	≈5 yrs	13%
Benson[45]	236	pN–	5 yrs	7.6%
	83	pN+	5 yrs	12.5%
Graversen[46]	648	1-2 nodes resected	6.5 yrs	10%
	793	3-4 nodes resected	6.5 yrs	5%
Sarrazin[75]	31	—	5 yrs	15%
Mazeron[76]	167	—	>5 yrs	10%
Partial Axillary Lymphadenectomy				
Benson[45]	243	pN–	5 yrs	2.9%
	75	pN+	5 yrs	12.5%
Graversen[46]	309	—	5 yrs	3%
Siegel[49]	259	—	22 mos	0.7%
Recht[77]	420	—	77 mos	2.1%
Total Axillary Lymphadenectomy				
Ball[22]	237	—	5 yrs	1.3%
Forrest[42]	79	—	≈5 yrs	4%
Kissin[44]	300	—	—	1%
NSABP B-04[47]	362	cN–	10 yrs	1.4%
	292	cN+	10 yrs	1.0%
Senofsky[51]	278	—	50 mos	0%
Veronesi[57]	701	—	7 yrs	< 1%
Kissin[61]	131	—	—	0%
Langlands[63]	256	—	5 yrs	2.7%
Mazeron[76†]	722	—	>5 yrs	1%
Axillary Radiotherapy Only				
NSABP B-04[47]	352	cN–	10 yrs	3.1%
	294	cN+	10 yrs	11.9%
Delouche[48]	294	cN–	>5 yrs	2.1%
Mazeron[76]	1527	—	>5 yrs	2%
Pierquin[78]	408	cN–	10 yrs	1.5%
Cabanes[79]	332	—	54 mos	2.1%
Axillary Surgery Plus Radiotherapy				
Forrest[41*]	64	—	10 yrs	16%
Benson[45*]	123	pN+	5 yrs	4.1%
Sarrazin[75*]	41	—	5 yrs	10%
Benson[45§]	132	pN+	5 yrs	2.3%
Dewar[62§]	132	—	5 yrs	0%
Recht[77§]	217	—	77 mos	0.9%
Cabanes[79§]	328	—	54 mos	0.9%
Fowble[80§]	914	—	40 mos	1.9%
Forrest[41¶]	66	—	10 yrs	1%
Delouche[48#]	116	—	>5 yrs	0%
Mazeron[76†]	937	—	>5 yrs	1%

cN– clinical node-negative	cN+ clinical node-positive	* node sampling plus radiotherapy
pN– pathological node-negative	pN+ pathological node-positive	§ PAL plus radiotherapy
¶ TAL plus radiotherapy	# PAL or TAL plus radiotherapy	

†   The axillary surgery in this series probably included both PAL and TAL; the patients were from a number of centers in several European countries, and the types of surgery performed were not clearly specified.

recurrence in less than 1% of patients undergoing TAL; because of this and the additional quantitative prognostic information provided, total lymphadenectomy remains their preferred treatment for the axillary nodes. In a prospective randomized trial of radical mastectomy (which of course includes TAL) versus total mastectomy plus axillary irradiation in patients with operable breast cancer, Langlands et al[63] reported 2.7% and 12.4% axillary failure rates (p < 0.0001), respectively, at a minimum followup of six years.

Whenever partial or subtotal resection of the axillary lymphatics is performed, there is an unavoidable risk of leaving residual disease in the axilla, as evidenced by the data on distribution of metastatic disease in the axilla (Tables 5-2 and 5-3). Apical and/or interpectoral metastases are present in 19% to 58% of pathological node-positive breast cancer patients (Table 5.2). In the University of Miami experience,[51,68] 31.5% of node-positive specimens were found to have metastatic disease in level III and/or Rotter's nodes, and in 10 cases these tumor deposits were evident on gross examination. Conservative axillary surgery therefore results in metastatic tumor being left in the axilla in a substantial minority of pathological node-positive patients, leaving them at higher risk for a clinically significant axillary relapse than would be the case with TAL.

When there is clinical or gross intraoperative evidence of level I or II nodal metastases at the time of surgery, there is little question that clearance of all of the axillary lymphatics is prudent.[21,76] In the University of Miami series, 43.8% of patients with gross level I and/or II disease were found to harbor further metastatic tumor in the apical and/or interpectoral nodes.[51,68] However, the absence of gross findings in the lower and mid-axilla should not be construed as assurance that there is little or no risk for involvement of the higher nodes. Of the 60 pathological node-positive axillae in the Miami series in which there was no gross evidence of disease in levels I and II, 15 or 25% had metastases in the apical or Rotter's nodes. A selective approach to the use of TAL based on the gross operative findings in levels

I and II would almost certainly have eventuated in clinical axillary relapse in a proportion of these patients. It is reiterated that with TAL, there were no axillary failures in these patients at 50 months' followup.

MORBIDITY OF AXILLARY INTERVENTION IN BREAST CANCER PATIENTS

FROZEN SHOULDER SYNDROME

Restriction of shoulder mobility is a relatively infrequent but highly significant sequela of axillary surgery and radiotherapy. The development of frozen shoulder syndrome following axillary lymphadenectomy can usually be vitiated by early, aggressive mobilization of the shoulder. For practical purposes, normal range of motion is restored in the ipsilateral shoulder joint by 6 months in the vast majority of patients.[81]

Clinically significant restriction of range of motion in the shoulder is more frequent when axillary staging surgery and axillary irradiation have been used in combination than when either is used separately. Patients in whom the axilla was treated by radiotherapy or, in the case of clinical node-positive patients, radiotherapy and limited axillary surgery by Pierquin et al[78] had minor deficits in range of motion in 5% to 10% of cases, generally related to radiation-induced pectoral muscle fibrosis. Rose et al[24] reported one patient with restricted shoulder range of motion among 178 in whom axillary management included axillary sampling plus radiotherapy. Dewar et al[62] reported range of motion deficits in 9% of patients undergoing limited axillary dissection plus radiation, and in only 1% of patients having only the limited axillary surgery (p < 0.0001). In a prospective randomized trial of lower axillary surgery versus surgery plus radiation, all three patients with shoulder mobility deficits were in the latter treatment arm.[75] Ryttov et al[82] reported a prospective trial in which a small number of patients with large breast cancers and/or extensive axillary involvement were randomized to lymphadenectomy or lymphadenectomy plus axillary irradiation. The incidence of shoulder mobility deficits was 12% in the surgery only arm and 38% in the group receiving radiotherapy. In a third group of patients with early stage breast cancer in whom axillary intervention was limited to surgery, the incidence of mobility problems was 4%.

BRACHIAL PLEXUS NEUROPATHY

Radiation-related brachial plexopathy develops in a small proportion of patients in whom the axillary and/or supraclavicular lymphatics have been irradiated.[31,83,84] This complication tends to present within the first three years following breast cancer treatment, which along with the absence of supraclavicular or distant metastases is an important differential feature vis-a-vis metastatic involvement of the brachial plexus by breast carcinoma. On occasion, surgical exploration with biopsy of the brachial plexus and surrounding soft tissue is required to establish the etiology (radiation versus carcinoma) of progressive upper extremity neurological dysfunction in breast cancer patients.[31] While infrequent, radiation-induced brachial plexus neuropathy is very difficult to treat.

Dewar et al[62] reported sensorimotor deficits in 2% of patients treated by axillary irradiation plus surgery as compared to 0.5% of those having axillary surgery only (p = 0.03). Sarrazin et al[75] in their prospective randomized trial of axillary surgery versus axillary surgery plus radiotherapy had one case of brachial plexopathy among patients in the latter treatment arm. Recht et al[77] reported brachial plexopathy in 2% of 896 patients treated with axillary plus supraclavicular radiotherapy as compared to 0.9% of 220 patients in whom the supraclavicular but not the axillary lymphatics were irradiated. None of the 508 patients in whom radiotherapy was confined to the breast developed this complication (p < 0.05 between the first and third groups).

RADIATION PNEUMONITIS

Recht et al[77] examined the incidence of symptomatic radiation pneumonitis by radiation treatment fields in the retrospective study from the Joint Center for Radiation Therapy. As with brachial plexopathy, the incidence of pneumonitis was highest in patients treated with axillary, supraclavicular and breast irradiation. The incidence of pneumonitis by radiotherapy treatment was 0.2% of patients treated to the breast only; 0.9% of patients treated to the breast and supraclavicular lymphatics and 1.6% of patients treated to all three areas. Axillary radiotherapy was administered mainly through an anterior field in these patients. In all cases, the pulmonary reaction to radiation exposure resolved without serious incident. Chemotherapy may have been contributory, although no supporting data were given.

IPSILATERAL UPPER EXTREMITY LYMPHEDEMA

The influence of axillary intervention on the incidence of clinically significant ipsilateral arm lymphedema is summarized in Table 5.5. This complication supervenes in up to 2.8% of patients undergoing only axillary biopsy or sampling,[39,40,44,45,62] 2.7% to 10% of patients in whom PAL has been performed,[45,48,49,61,82] 4.8% to 8% of patients treated by TAL[21,22,44,51,57,61] and 2% to 8.3% of those who undergo axillary irradiation only, without surgical staging.[48,59,61,78,84] On the whole, the incidence of ipsilateral upper extremity edema is modest and its severity is within tolerable limits when surgery or radiation are used alone. However, when axillary surgery and irradiation are used in combination, there is a 3- to 10-fold increase in the incidence of subsequent arm lymphedema.[48,51,59,61,62,78,82,83]

In the University of Miami experience, arm lymphedema developed in 9.4% of cases.[51,68] Clinically problematic lymphedema (i.e. persistent, significant swelling for which an external compression stocking or the use of a lymphedema pump was required, or lymphedema complicated by recurring lymphangitis) occurred in 5.4%. However, among patients in whom the regional lymphatics were not irradiated, the overall and clinically significant incidences of lymphedema were only 6% and 3.7%, respectively. These figures are very much in line with those reported for PAL. There is little evidence to suggest that, in performing an axillary lymphadenectomy, resection of the

Table 5.5 Incidence of ipsilateral upper extremity lymphedema following treatment of the axilla in breast cancer patients

Axillary Intervention	No. Patients	No. with Lymphedema		Followup
Axillary Sampling				
Benson[45]	463	13	(2.8%)	2-7 yrs
Larson[59]	191*	12	(6.3%)	45 mos
Carabell[60]	84*	0	(0%)	>1 yr
Kissin[61]	17	0	(0%)	>1 yr
	22*	2	(9.1%)	>1 yr
Dewar[62†]	423	6	(2.0%)	78 mos
	164*	33	(20.0%)	78 mos
Partial Axillary Lymphadenectomy				
Benson[45]	497	25	(5.0%)	2-7 yrs
Siegel[49]	259	7	(2.7%)	27 mos
Larson[59]	49*	18	(36.7%)	45 mos
Kissin[61]	94	7	(7.4%)	>1 yr
	47*	18	(38.3%)	>1 yr
Ryttov[82]	40	4	(10.0%)	42 mos
Beadle[85]	109*	13	(11.9%)	30 mos
Total Axillary Lymphadenectomy				
Danforth[21]	136	7	(5.6%)	not given
Ball[22]	50	3	(6.0%)	5 yrs
Kissin[44]	50	4	(8.0%)	5 yrs
Senofsky[51]	217	13	(6.0%)	50 mos
	61*	13	(21.3%)	50 mos
Veronesi[57]	352‡	11	(3.1%)	7 yrs
	349§	23	(6.6%)	7 yrs
Radiotherapy Alone				
Delouche[48]	294	10	(3.4%)	11 yrs
Larson[59]	235	10	(4.0%)	45 mos
Kissin[61]	12	1	(8.3%)	>1 yr
Pierquin[78]	408	—	(< 5%)	10 yrs
Beadle[85]	96	2	(2.1%)	30 mos

In this Table, the axillary therapies employed in these series were categorized by the description of the treatment or operation given in the Methods section of each publication.

* These patients received postoperative adjuvant axillary radiotherapy as well.
† Two-thirds of these patients had lower axillary sampling, one-third PAL.
‡ Treated with conservative surgery, total axillary lymphadenectomy and radiotherapy.
§ Treated by radical mastectomy.

Adapted from Moffat FL, et al. J Surg Oncol 1992; 51:8-13 © 1992, Wiley-Liss

apical and interpectoral nodes significantly adds to the likelihood of a patient developing this complication. Moreover, resection of these nodes extends operative time by no more than 5 to 10 minutes, and requires no special surgical expertise.

Irradiated patients had a five-fold higher incidence of upper extremity edema in the University of Miami series, a highly significant difference (Fig. 5.2). In that PAL and especially TAL are so highly effective in preventing axillary relapse when used alone, axillary irradiation can add little or nothing in terms of disease control or survival,[26,32-36,47,50,63,67,82,85-90] but greatly increases the prospects for arm lymphedema.[48,51,59,61,62,82] Irradiation of the ipsilateral breast in patients undergoing breast-conserving therapy has not been causally linked to the development of upper extremity lymphedema.[51,61]

It is well recognized by general, oncological and vascular surgeons that skeletonization of the axillary vein in the course of performing an axillary dissection greatly increases the prospects for long term problems with chronic upper extremity swelling.[33,61] In that there are few or no lymph nodes above the axillary vein, and that there is a functionally significant plexus of lymphatic vessels in the vein adventitia and immediately adjacent normal tissues, there is nothing to be gained and much to be lost by extensively dissecting the tissues anterior and superior to the vein. Having acknowledged this truth, one of the basic technical principles of vascular surgery is that the safest plane of dissection in the vicinity of a large vessel is on its adventitial surface.[10]

Therefore, the best course is to dissect the axillary fat pad off the inferior adventitial surface of the vein, and to leave the anterior, posterior and superior surfaces of the vein and adjacent tissues undisturbed.

Some have advocated limited lymphadenectomies or node sampling operations in which no formal attempt is made to visualize the axillary vein during the procedure. In three breast cancer series in which such axillary surgery was performed, 0.6% to 7.2% of patients developed axillary vein thrombosis perioperatively,[24,49,60] a complication which of course puts the patient at risk for upper extremity lymphedema due to the combined venous and lymphatic compromise. Axillary vein thrombosis in this setting probably occurred as a result of unrecognized traction injuries or other surgical trauma to the undissected vein. Complications of this nature are extremely unusual when the vein has been visualized and the axillary contents carefully dissected off its inferior surface.

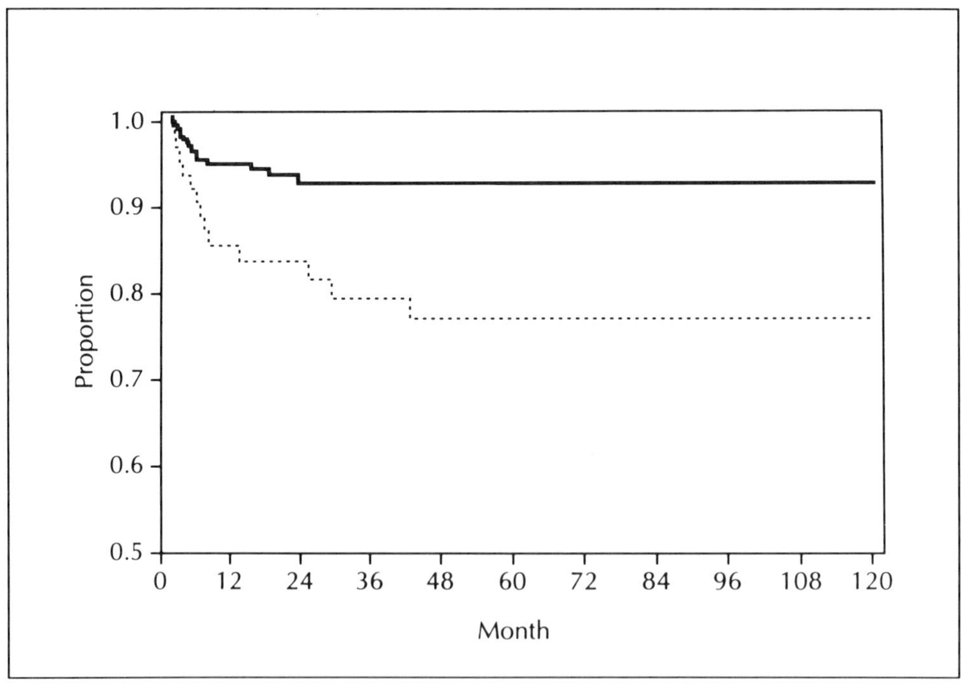

Fig. 5.2. Proportions of irradiated (dotted line) and nonirradiated (solid line) patients in the University of Miami series,[51] estimated by the Kaplan-Meier method, which remained free of ipsilateral upper extremity lymphedema following total axillary lymphadenectomy. Of the 61 irradiated patients, 13 developed arm lymphedema as compared to 13 of 217 nonirradiated patients (X^2_{1df} = 11.44, p < 0.001). Reproduced with permission from Senofsky GM, et al. Arch Surg 1991; 126:1336-1342. © 1991, American Medical Association.

AXILLARY LYMPHADENECTOMY AND LYMPHEDEMA OF THE CONSERVED BREAST

This has been addressed in detail in the preceeding chapter. Briefly, postoperative edema in the conserved breast has been correlated with axillary dissection, but the effect is modest and subsides over the first several months to two years of followup.[85,91]

MANAGEMENT OF THE AXILLARY LYMPHATICS

SUMMARY OF PRESENT STATUS

Of the currently available axillary management options in breast cancer patients, PAL (incorporating Berg's levels I and II) and TAL are much superior to lesser surgical procedures for staging the axilla. As noted, the current status of systemic adjuvant therapy is such that detailed and precise information regarding axillary lymph node status is essential for appropriate selection of patients for the various types of systemic cytotoxic therapy. Therefore, a large number of lymph nodes must be resected for histopathological examination. TAL and level I and II PAL meet these stringent requirements while axillary node sampling and biopsy clearly do not.

Objections to subtotal or total axillary dissections on the basis of excessive morbidity, particularly with reference to ipsilateral upper extremity lymphedema, are largely unfounded. Provided the regional lymphatics are not irradiated, the incidence of lymphedema following level I, level I and II, or total axillary lymphadenectomy is quite acceptable; in fact, the incidence of lymphedema associated with TAL is essentially the same as that of level I and II PAL. TAL requires minimal additional surgical effort or risk as compared to PAL, eliminates surgical staging error altogether when properly performed, and most effectively abrogates the risk of axillary relapse. For these reasons, TAL is the preferred approach to the axilla in a number of institutions.[22,29,30,44,51,57,61,63,68]

Irradiation of the axilla, especially in clinical node-negative patients, is also highly effective in preventing axillary relapse. The incidence of complications is very low as long as radiotherapy is not combined with axillary surgery other than perhaps diagnostic biopsy.[59,60] However, it is no longer sufficient to simply determine whether pathological nodal status is positive or negative, or to routinely disregard nodal status altogether, and these circumstances are likely to endure for the foreseeable future. For this reason, the routine use of axillary radiotherapy alone or with axillary biopsy should no longer be included among the optimal treatment approaches to the axilla in early breast cancer. However, axillary radiation therapy remains a very safe and efficacious alternative for breast cancer patients who for any reason (medical risks, physical infirmity, refusal of surgery or general anaesthesia, etc.) are not candidates for axillary lymphadenectomy.

As axillary recurrence is very unusual following level I and II PAL or TAL, adjuvant axillary irradiation used in combination with these procedures can provide no measurable clinical benefit. Moreover, the risk of disabling lymphedema increases dramatically when lymphadenectomy and axillary radiotherapy are used in combination. Irradiation of the axilla should be scrupulously avoided in patients undergoing PAL or TAL for early breast cancer.

FUTURE PROSPECTS

With the rapid progress in development of systemic adjuvant therapy, it is possible that current requirements for precise quantitative information on axillary node status will lessen or perhaps disappear entirely. As the complication rate and mortality of bone marrow transplantation decline, radical chemotherapy may become a viable or even the preferred option for all node-positive patients. It is not inconceivable that limited axillary staging procedures might once again provide sufficient information for decision-making vis-`a-vis systemic cytotoxic therapy.

Recent diagnostic developments hold forth the distinct possibility that reliable elucidation of axillary nodal status might soon be possible without having to resort to lymphadenectomy on a routine basis. The advent of radioimmunoscintigraphy has made possible the imaging of lymph node micrometastases in patients with colorectal cancer,[92-94] melanoma,[95] prostatic carcinoma[96] and breast cancer,[97-99] and other tumors. This technology is based on the use of radiolabeled monoclonal antibodies with specificity for tumor antigens. The radioimmunoconjugate targets and binds to tumor cells, and external scintigraphy can then image deposits of tumor as small as 0.5 cm. The tumor can also be localized by intraoperative use of a gamma radiation detection probe. Although this diagnostic modality is in its infancy, there is much optimism about its potential value in decision-making in oncology and in breast cancer in particular. An obvious application would be the use of these techniques to determine noninvasively whether the axillary lymphatics in patients with early breast cancer are involved by tumor. Lymphadenectomy could then be performed only in those with demonstrable nodal involvement.

The older "sentinel node" concept is being revisited as a promising alternative to routine axillary lymphadenectomy. Morton et al[100] injected vital dyes into primary cutaneous melanoma sites in an effort to identify the sentinel node in the regional lymphatic basin, which the melanoma would therefore be most likely to involve first if metastasis via the lymphatics had already occurred. After injection of the dye, an incision was made over the regional nodes and thin skin flaps were raised to allow direct visualization of the dye-filled lymphatic vessels coming from the primary tumor site. The lymphatics were then traced to the sentinel "blue" node, which was then resected and submitted for histopathological examination. Sentinel nodes were identified in 147 of 237 regional lymph node basins in melanoma patients, and metastases were identified in 40. The false-negative rate with this technique was less than 1%, suggesting that this may be useful in determining which clinical node-negative melanoma patients should undergo elective regional lymphadenectomy.

Krag and co-workers[101-103] have modified this technique, substituting [99m]technetium-sulphur colloid for the vital dye. A gamma detection probe is used to localize the senti-

nel node which is then excised through an incision placed directly over it. This modification avoids the necessity for a skin flap, which has been a significant source of complications with the vital dye technique.[100] Following successful preclinical studies in cats,[101] this method has been used in clinical node-negative melanoma[102] and breast cancer patients.[103] In the breast cancer study,[103] 22 consecutive breast cancer patients were studied after injection of 0.4 mCi [99m]technetium sulphur colloid around the periphery of the primary cancer. The gamma detection probe detected sentinel nodes in 18 patients, and in the seven patients who proved to be pathologically node-positive, the sentinel nodes were positive in every case. In three of these patients, the identified sentinel node was the only involved node in the axilla. These results are highly encouraging; if this methodology proves to have a negligible false-negative rate, a selective approach to axillary lymphadenectomy might then become feasible. The available data strongly suggest that this technique would prove far superior to the older random or surgically directed sampling procedures.[39-45]

As discussed in previous chapters, there is a prodigious research effort underway to elucidate factors such as oncogene products, histochemical or flow cytometry parameters which would accurately predict breast cancer dissemination. As of this date, pathological axillary node status remains the most significant predictor of adverse outcome in breast cancer patients.

References

1. Carter CL, Allen C, Henson DE. Relation of tumor size, lymph node status, and survival in 24,740 breast cancer cases. Cancer 1989; 63:181-187.

2. Fisher B, Ravdin RG, Ausman RK, et al. Surgical adjuvant chemotherapy in cancer of the breast: results of a decade of cooperative investigation. Ann Surg 1968; 168:337-356.

3. Fisher B, Bauer M, Wickerham DL, et al. Relation of number of positive axillary nodes to the prognosis of patients with primary breast cancer. An NSABP update. Cancer 1983; 52:1551-1557.

4. Fisher B, Carbone P, Economou SG, et al. L-phenylalanine mustard (L-PAM) in the management of primary breast cancer. A report of early findings. New Engl J Med 1975; 292:117-122.

5. Bonadonna G, Brusamolino E, Valagussa P, et al. Combination chemotherapy as an adjuvant treatment for operable breast cancer. New Engl J Med 1976; 294:405-410.

6. Nolvadex Adjuvant Trial Organization. Controlled trial of tamoxifen as a single agent in the management of early breast cancer. Analysis at eight years. Br J Cancer 1988; 57:608-611.

7. Ludwig Breast Cancer Study Group. Randomised trial of chemo-endocrine therapy, endocrine therapy, and mastectomy alone in postmenopausal patients with operable breast cancer and axillary node metastasis. Lancet 1984; 1:1256-1260.

8. Early Breast Cancer Trialists' Collaborative Group. Systemic treatment of early breast cancer by hormonal, cytotoxic, or immune therapy. 133 randomised trials involving 31,000 recurrences and 24,000 deaths among 75,000 women. Lancet 1992; 339: 1-15, 71-85.

9. Fisher ER, Costantino J, Fisher B, et al. Pathologic findings from the National Surgical Adjuvant Breast Project (Protocol 4). Discriminants for 15-year survival. Cancer 1993; 71:2141-2150.

10. Fisher ER, Anderson S, Redmond C, Fisher B. Pathologic findings from the National Surgical Adjuvant Breast Project Protocol B-06. Cancer 1993; 71:2507-2514.

11. Meropol NJ, Stadtmauer EA. High-dose chemotherapy with autologous stem cell support for breast cancer. Oncology 1992; 6:53-63.

12. Bonadonna G, Valagussa P. Adjuvant systemic therapy for resectable breast cancer. J Clin Oncol 1985; 3:259-275.

13. Bonadonna G, Valagussa P. Dose-intense adjuvant therapy of high risk breast cancer. J Natl Cancer Inst 1990; 82:542-543.

14. Gianni AM, Siena S, Bregi M, et al. Growth factor-supported high dose sequential adjuvant chemotherapy in breast cancer with more than 10 positive nodes. Proc Amer Soc Clin Oncol 1992; 11:60 (Abstr).

15. Peters WP, Ross M, Vendenberg J, et al. High dose alkylating agents and autologous bone marrow support (ABMT) for Stage II/III breast cancer involving 10 or more axillary nodes. Proc Amer Soc Clin Oncol 1992; 11:58 (Abstr).

16. Fisher B, Wolmark N, Bauer M, Redmond C, Gebhardt M. The accuracy of clinical nodal staging and of limited axillary dissection as a determinant of histological nodal status in carcinoma of the breast. Surg Gynecol Obstet 1981; 152:765-772.

17. Fisher B, Redmond C, Dimitrov NV, et al. A randomized clinical trial evaluating sequential methotrexate and fluorouracil in the treatment of patients with node-negative breast cancer who have estrogen-receptor-negative tumors. New Engl J Med 1989; 320: 473-478.

18. Fisher B, Costantino J, Redmond C, et al. A randomized clinical trial evaluating tamoxifen in the treatment of patients with node-negative breast cancer who have estrogen-receptor-positive tumors. New Engl JK Med 1989; 320:479-484.

19. Mansour EG, Gray R, Shatila AH, et al. Efficacy of adjuvant chemotherapy in high-risk node-negative breast cancer. An Intergroup study. New Engl J Med 1989; 320:485-490.

20. The Ludwig Breast Cancer Study Group. Prolonged disease-free survival after one course of perioperative adjuvant chemotherapy for node-negative breast cancer. New Engl J Med 1989; 320:491-496.

21. Danforth DN Jr., Findlay PA, McDonald HD, et al. Complete axillary lymph node dissection for Stage I-II carcinoma of the breast. J Clin Oncol 1986; 4:655-662.

22. Ball ABS, Fish S, Waters R, Thomas JM. Radical axillary dissection in the staging and treatment of breast cancer. Ann Roy Coll Surg Engl 1992; 74:126-129.

23. Lin PP, Allison DC, Wainstock J, et al. Impact of axillary lymph node dissection on the therapy of breast cancer patients. J Clin Oncol 1993; 11:1536-1544.

24. Rose CM, Botnick LE, Weinstein M, et al. Axillary sampling in the definitive treatment of breast cancer by radiation therapy and lumpectomy. Int J Radiat Oncol Biol Phys 1983; 9:339-344.

25. Cutler SJ, Axtell LM, Schottenfeld D, Farrow JH. Clinical assessment of lymph nodes in carcinoma of the breast. Surg Gynecol Obstet 1970; 131:41-52.

26. Davies GC, Millis RR, Hayward JL. Assessment of axillary lymph node status. Ann Surg 1980; 192:148-151.

27. Chevinsky AH, Ferrara J, James AG, et al. Prospective evaluation of clinical and pathologic detection of axillary metastases in patients with carcinoma of the breast. Surgery 1990; 108:612-618.

28. Kitchen PRB, McLennan R, Mursell A. Node-positive breast cancer: a comparison of clinical and pathological findings and assessment of axillary clearance. Aust NZ J Surg 1980; 50:580-583.

29. Veronesi U, Rilke F, Luini A, et al. Distribution of axillary node metastases by level of invasion. An analysis of 539 cases. Cancer 1987; 59:682-687.

30. Veronesi U, Luini A, Galimberti S, et al. Extent of metastatic axillary involvement in 1446 cases of breast cancer. Eur J Surg Oncol 1990; 16:127-133.

31. Bagley FH, Walsh JW, Cady B, et al. Carcinomatous versus radiation-induced brachial plexus neuropathy in breast cancer. Cancer 1978; 41:2154-2157.

32. Fisher ER, Palekar A, Rockette H, et al. Pathologic findings from the National Surgical Adjuvant Breast Project (Protocol No. 4). V. Significance of axillary nodal micro- and macrometastases. Cancer 1978; 42:2032-2038.

33. Recht A, Connolly JL, Schnitt SJ, et al. Conservative surgery and radiation therapy for early breast cancer: results, controversies, and unsolved problems. Semin Oncol 1986; 13:434-449.

34. Huvos AG, Hutter RVP, Berg JW. Significance of axillary macrometastases and micrometastases in mammary cancer. Ann Surg 1971; 173:44-46.

35. Fisher ER, Swamidoss S, Lee CH, et al. Detection and significance of occult axillary node metastases in patients with invasive breast cancer. Cancer 1978; 42:2025-2031.

36. Rosen PP, Saigo PE, Braun DW, et al. Axillary micro- and macrometastases in breast cancer. Ann Surg 1981; 194:585-591.

37. Fisher ER, Gregorio RM, Redmond C, Kim WS, Fisher B. Pathologic findings from the National Surgical Adjuvant Breast Project (Protocol No. 4). III. The significance of extranodal extension of axillary metastases. Amer J Clin Pathol 1976; 65:439-444.

38. Donegan WL, Stine SB, Samter TG. Implications of extracapsular nodal metastases for treatment and prognosis of breast cancer. Cancer 1993; 72:778-782.

39. Steele RJC, Forrest APM, Gibson T, et al. The efficacy of lower axillary sampling in obtaining lymph node status in breast cancer: a controlled randomized trial. Br J Surg 1985; 72:368-369.

40. Forrest APM, Roberts MM, Cant ELM, et al. Simple mastectomy and pectoral node biopsy: the Cardiff-St. Mary's trial. World J Surg 1977; 1:320-323.

41. Forrest APM, Stewart HJ, Roberts MM, Steele RJC. Simple mastectomy and axillary node sampling (pectoral node biopsy) in the management of primary breast cancer. Ann Surg 1982; 196:371-378.

42. Cant ELM, Shivas AA, Forrest APM. Lymph-node biopsy during simple mastectomy. Lancet 1975; 2:995-997.

43. Forrest APM, Roberts MM, Cant ELM, Shivas AA. Simple mastectomy and pectoral node biopsy. Br J Surg 1976; 63:569-575.

44. Kissin MW, Thompson EM, Price AB, et al. The inadequacy of axillary node sampling in breast cancer. Lancet 1982; 2:1210-1212.

45. Benson EA, Thorogood J. The effect of surgical technique on local recurrence rates following mastectomy. Eur J Surg Oncol 1986; 12:267-271.

46. Graversen HP, Blichert-Toft M, Andersen JA, et al. Breast cancer: risk of axillary recurrence in node-negative patients following partial dissection of the axilla. Eur J Surg Oncol 1988; 14: 407-412.

47. Fisher B, Redmond C, Fisher ER, et al. Ten-year results of a randomized clinical trial comparing radical mastectomy and total mastectomy with and without radiation. New Engl J Med 1985; 312:674-681.

48. Delouche G, Bachelot F, Premont M, Kurtz JM. Conservation treatment of early breast cancer: long term results and complications. Int J Radiat Oncol Biol Phys 1987; 13:29-34.

49. Siegel BM, Mayzel KA, Love SM. Level I and II axillary dissection in the treatment of early-stage breast cancer: an analysis of 259 consecutive patients. Arch Surg 1990; 125:1144-1147.

50. Fisher B, Wolmark N, Bauer M, et al. The accuracy of clinical nodal staging and of limited axillary dissection as a determinant of histologic nodal status in carcinoma of the breast. Surg Gynecol Obstet 1981; 152:764-772.

51. Senofsky GM, Moffat FL, Davis K, et al. Total axillary lymphadenectomy in the management of breast cancer. Arch Surg 1991; 126:1336-1342.

52. Rosen PP, Lesser ML, Kinne DW, Beattie EJ. Discontinuous or "skip" metastases in breast carcinoma. Analysis of 1228 axillary dissections. Ann Surg 1983; 197:276-283.

53. Schwartz GF, D'Ugo DM, Rosenberg AL. Extent of axillary dissection preceeding irradiation for carcinoma of the breast. Arch Surg 1986; 121:1395-1398.

54. Pigott J, Nichols R, Maddox WA, Balch CM. Metastases to the upper levels of the axillary nodes in carcinoma of the breast and its implications for node sampling procedures. Surg Gynecol Obstet 1984; 158:255-259.

55. Attiyeh FF, Jensen M, Huvos AG, Fracchia A. Axillary micrometastasis and macrometastasis in carcinoma of the breast. Surg Gynecol Obstet 1977; 144:839-842.

56. Smith JA, Gamez-Araujo JJ, Gallager HS, et al. Carcinoma of the breast. Analysis of total lymph node involvement versus level of metastasis. Cancer 1977; 39:527-533.

57. Veronesi U, Saccozzi R, Del Vecchio M, et al. Comparing radical mastectomy with quadrantectomy, axillary dissection and radiotherapy in patients with small cancers of the breast. New Engl J Med 1981; 305:6-11.

58. Boova RS, Bonanni R, Rosato FE. Patterns of axillary nodal involvement in breast cancer. Predictability of level one dissection. Ann Surg 1982; 196:642-644.

59. Larson D, Weinstein M, Goldberg I, et al. Edema of the arm as a function of the extent of axillary surgery in patients with Stage I - II carcinoma of the breast treated with primary radiotherapy. Int J Radiat Oncol Biol Phys 1986; 12:1575-1582.

60. Carabell SC, Richter MP, Bryan JH, et al. Radiation therapy as an alternative to mastectomy for breast cancer - the role of axillary sampling. Int J Radiat Oncol Biol Phys 1981; 7:31-32.

61. Kissin MW, Querci della Rovere G, Easton D, Westbury G. Risk of lymphedema following the treatment of breast cancer. Br J Surg 1986; 73:580-584.

62. Dewar JA, Sarrazin D, Benhamou E, et al. Management of the axilla in conservatively treated breast cancer: 592 patients treated at Institut Gustave-Roussy. Int J Radiat Oncol Biol Phys 1987; 13:475-481.

63. Langlands AO, Prescott RJ, Hamilton T. A clinical trial in the management of operable breast cancer. Br J Surg 1980; 67:170-174.

64. Berg JW. The significance of axillary node levels in the study of breast carcinoma. Cancer 1955; 4:776-778.

65. Temple WJ, Ketcham AS. Preservation of the intercostobrachial nerves during axillary dissection for breast cancer. Amer J Surg 1985; 150:585-588.

66. Merson M, Pirovano C, Balzarini A, et al. The preservation of minor pectoralis muscle in axillary dissection for breast cancer: functional and cosmetic evaluation. Eur J Surg Oncol 1992; 18:215-218.

67. Cody HS, Egeli RA, Urban JA. Rotter's node metastases. Therapeutic and prognostic considerations in early breast cancer. Ann Surg 1984; 199:266-270.

68. Moffat FL, Senofsky GM, Davis K, et al. Axillary node dissection for early breast cancer: some is good, but all is better. J Surg Oncol 1992; 51:8-13.

69. Gaglia P, Bussone R, Caldarola B, et al. The correlation between the spread of metastases by level in the axillary nodes and disease-free survival in breast cancer. A multifactorial analysis. Eur J Cancer Clin Oncol 1987; 23:849-854.

70. Toma S, Leonessa F, Romanini A, et al. Predictive value of some clinical and pathological parameters on upper level axillary node involvement in breast cancer. Anticancer Res 1991; 11:1439-1444.

71. Barth RJ, Danforth DN Jr., Venzon DJ, et al. Level of axillary involvement by lymph node metastases from breast cancer is not an independent predictor of survival. Arch Surg 1991; 126:574-577.

72. Kiricuta CI, Tausch J. A mathematical model of axillary lymph node involvement based on 1446 complete axillary dissections in patients with breast carcinoma. Cancer 1992; 69:2496-2501.

73. Axelsson CK, Mouridsen HT, Zedeler K, et al. Axillary dissection of level I and II lymph nodes is important in breast cancer classification. Eur J Cancer 1992; 28A:1415-1418.

74. Kjærgaard J, Blichert-Toft M, Andersen JA, et al. Probability of false negative nodal staging in conjunction with partial axillary dissection in breast cancer. Br J Surg 1985; 72:365-367.

75. Sarrazin D, Lê M, Rouësse J, et al. Conservative treatment versus mastectomy in breast cancer tumors with macroscopic diameter of 20 millimeters or less. The experience of the Institut Gustave-Roussy. Cancer 1984; 53:1209-1213.

76. Mazeron JJ, Otmezguine Y, Huart J, Pierquin B. Conservative treatment of breast cancer: results of management of axillary lymph node area in 3353 patients. Lancet 1985; 2:1387.

77. Recht A, Pierce SM, Abner A, et al. Regional nodal failure after conservative surgery and radiotherapy for early-stage breast carcinoma. J Clin Oncol 1991; 9:988-996.

78. Pierquin B, Otmezguine Y, Lobo PA. Conservative management of breast cancer. the Créteil experience. Acta Radiol Oncol 1983; 22:101-107.

79. Cabanes PA, Salmon RJ, Vilcoq JR, et al. Value of axillary dissection in addition to lumpectomy and radiotherapy in early breast cancer. Lancet 1992; 339:1245-1248.

80. Fowble B, Solin LJ, Schultz DJ, Goodman RL. Frequency, sites of relapse, and outcome of regional node failures following conservative surgery and radiation for early breast cancer. Int J Radiat Oncol Biol Phys 1989; 17:703-710.

81. Hladiuk M, Huchcroft S, Temple W, Schnurr BE. Arm function after axillary dissection for breast cancer: a pilot study to provide parameter estimates. J Surg Oncol 1992; 50:47-52.

82. Ryttov N, Holm NV, Qvist N, Blichert-Toft M. Influence of adjuvant irradiation on the development of late arm lymphedema and impaired shoulder mobility after mastectomy for carcinoma of the breast. Acta Oncol 1988; 27:667-671.

83. Match RM. Radiation-induced brachial plexus paralysis. Arch Surg 1975; 110:384-386.

84. Salner AL, Botnick LE, Herzog AG, et al. Reversible brachial plexopathy following primary radiation therapy for breast cancer. Cancer Treat Rep 1981; 65:797-801.

85. Beadle GF, Silver B, Botnick L, et al. Cosmetic results following primary radiation therapy for early breast cancer. Cancer 1984; 54:2911-2914.

86. Fisher B, Slack NH, Cavanaugh PJ, et al. Postoperative radiotherapy in the treatment of breast cancer: results of the NSABP clinical trial. Ann Surg 1970; 172:711-732.

87. Fisher B, Montague E, Redmond C, et al. Comparison of radical mastectomy with alternative treatments for breast cancer. A first report of results from a prospective randomized clinical trial. Cancer 1977; 39:2827-2839.

88. Fisher B, Wolmark N, Redmond C, et al. Findings from NSABP B-04: comparison of radical mastectomy with alternative treatments. II. The clinical and biological significance of medial-central breast cancers. Cancer 1981; 48:1863-1872.

89. Fisher B, Montague E, Redmond C, et al. Findings from NSABP Protocol No. 4— comparison of radical mastectomy with alternative treatments for primary breast cancer. I. Radiation compliance and its relation to treatment outcome. Cancer 1980; 46:1-13.

90. Clark RM, Wilkinson RH, Miceli PN, MacDonald WD. Breast cancer. Experiences with conservation therapy. Amer J Clin Oncol 1987; 10:461-468.

91. Clarke D, Martinez A, Cox RS, Goffinet DR. Breast edema following staging axillary node dissection in patients with breast carcinoma treated by radical radiotherapy. Cancer 1982; 49:2295-2299.

92. Moffat FL, Vargas-Cuba RD, Serafini AN, et al. Radioimmunodetection of colorectal carcinoma using technetium 99m-labeled Fab' fragments of the IMMU-4 anti-carcinoembryonic antigen monoclonal antibody. Cancer 1994; 73: 836-845.

93. Kuhn JA, Corbisiero RM, Buras RR, et al. Intraoperative gamma detection probe with presurgical antibody imaging in colon cancer. Arch Surg 1991; 126:1398-1403.

94. Arnold MW, Schneebaum S, Berens A, et al. Radioimmunoguided surgery challenges traditional decision making in patients with primary colorectal cancer. Surgery 1992; 112:624-630.

95. Blend MJ, Ronan SG, Salk DJ, Das Gupta TK. Role of technetium 99m-labeled monoclonal antibody in the management of melanoma patients. J Clin Oncol 1992; 10:1330-1337.

96. Badalament RA, Burgers JK, Petty LR, et al. Radioimmunoguided radical prostatectomy and lymphadenectomy. Cancer 1993; 71:2268-2275.

97. Nieroda CA, Mojzisik C, Sardi A, et al. Staging of carcinoma of the breast using a hand-held gamma detecting probe and monoclonal antibody B72.3. Surg Gynecol Obstet 1989; 169:35-40.

98. Athanassiou A, Pectasides D, Pateniotis K, et al. Immunoscintigraphy with ^{131}I-labelled HMFG$_2$ F(ab')$_2$ in the preoperative detection of clinical and subclinical lymph node metastases in breast cancer patients. Int J Cancer 1988; Suppl 3:89-95.

99. Tjandra JJ, Sacks NPM, Thompson CH, et al. The detection of axillary lymph node metastases from breast cancer by radiolabelled monoclonal antibodies: a prospective study. Br J Cancer 1989; 59:296-302.

100. Morton DL, Wen D-R, Wong JH, et al. Technical details of intraoperative lymphatic mapping for early stage melanoma. Arch Surg 1992; 127:392-399.

101. Alex JC, Krag DN. Gamma-probe guided localization of lymph nodes. Surg Oncol 1993; 2:137-143.

102. Alex JC, Weaver DL, Fairbank JT, Rankin BS, Krag DN. Gamma-probeguided lymph node localization in malignant melanoma. Surg Oncol 1993; 2:303-308.

103. Krag DN, Weaver DL, Alex JC, Fairbank JT. Surgical resection and radiolocalization of the sentinel lymph node in breast cancer using a gamma probe. Surg Oncol 1993; 2:335-340.

CHAPTER 6

DUCTAL CARCINOMA IN SITU

The clinical management of patients with noninvasive breast cancer continues to be a major controversy in clinical oncology. The recent dramatic increase in incidence of preinvasive breast disease is the result of the widespread practice of mammographic screening as well as heightened awareness and more accurate diagnosis of these lesions by surgical pathologists.

Preinvasive breast cancer was first described in 1913 by MacCarty.[1] In 1932, Broders[2] defined carcinoma in situ as a condition in which malignant epithelial cells are identified in positions previously occupied by their normal ancestors, but which have not migrated beyond the normal epithelial basement membrane. Foote and Stewart further documented and characterized in situ breast neoplasia with the first description of lobular carcinoma in situ,[3] a comparison study of cancerous and noncancerous breast tissue,[4] and a classification of preinvasive and infiltrating carcinoma of the breast.[5] Subsequent work has led to the currently held biological precept that, in the transformation of normal epithelial elements into invasive and metastasizing neoplastic cells, several intermediate cytological states exist.[6,7] Ductal proliferation or hyperplasia in response to a variety of known and as yet unknown stimuli are thought to evolve through the ductal carcinoma in situ (DCIS) state into invasive neoplasia. Progression of normal ductal cells through this morphological continuum occurs over time, but may not run its full course to neoplasia. This process of malignant transformation may only be truly irreversible either when the cytological criteria of neoplasia are met, or when cytologically malignant cells acquire the capacity to invade and metastasize.

In situ cancer cells are cytologically indistinguishable from those infiltrating the surrounding normal breast parenchyma.[2] However, as with invasive malignant neoplasms in other organ systems, intraductal carcinoma of the breast is not invariably observed in every patient diagnosed with infiltrating breast cancer. Conversely, as many as 30% to 40% of in situ cancers occur in association with invasive carcinoma.

TISSUE DIAGNOSIS OF NONPALPABLE BREAST LESIONS

Historically, most DCIS lesions were extensive, palpable tumors, or presented as Paget's disease of the nipple. Presently, the great majority of intraductal carcinomas are nonpalpable, being discovered mostly by mammography. Most nonpalpable in situ lesions present on mammography as clustered or segmental linear microcalcifications, with or without an associated soft tissue density, in a background of fibrocystic change. DCIS is encountered as an incidental finding in up to 10% of benign breast biopsies.

Mammographic detection of subclinical breast abnormalities necessitated the development and widespread application of the needle localization breast biopsy (NLBB) technique and, more recently, computerized stereotactic core needle breast biopsy (SCNB) technology. Excisional biopsy of nonpalpable or clinically indistinct breast lesions using preoperative needle localization for guidance of the surgeon (Fig. 6.1A) requires close cooperation between radiologist and surgeon. These are demanding procedures for the surgeon, who must be able to conceptualize in three dimensions when interpreting the preoperative needle localization mammogram with the radiologist. Because of the spatial uncertainty inherent in the NLBB technique, a larger amount of tissue is often excised than for palpable lesions; this apparent paradox relates to the necessity to resect more tissue simply to minimize the chance of missing the lesion in question. In some cases, the surgeon is able to palpate the lesion as it is approached in the course of the biopsy. This gives added assurance that it has been identified and removed. In any event, a specimen mammogram is performed immediately following excision of the tissue to ascertain that the mammographic abnormality of interest has indeed been removed, and to assist the pathologist in identifying the lesion within the submitted tissue (Fig. 6.1B).

Unfortunately, even experienced radiologists and surgeons will inevitably miss mammographic abnormalities altogether with NLBB, on occasion. Rusnak et al[8] reported six cases among 200 (3%) in which the mammographic abnormality of interest was missed by NLBB. Specimen mammography minimizes but does not preclude this possibility which, in the present litiginous climate, often has legal ramifications. For this reason, a mammogram of the biopsied breast four months postoperatively (or after the early cicatricial reaction in the biopsy wound has subsided) is mandatory when a benign diagnosis has been made. This inherent limitation in the NLBB technique should motivate surgeons to inform their patients preoperatively of the small likelihood of missing the mammographic abnormality of interest.

Stereotactic techniques have made feasible the use of fine needle aspiration cytology and core needle biopsy for diagnosis of nonpalpable mammographic abnormalities. SCNB produces minimal cutaneous and parenchymal cicatricial reaction, and therefore does not interfere with subsequent surveillance of the biopsied breast. It is also significantly less expensive than NLBB.[9]

SCNB is performed with the patient prone, the breast protruding through an aperture in the table and immobilized in a mammographic compression device. The abnormality of interest is identified on mammography and positioned within the localization window (Fig. 6.2A), and stereoscopic views are then obtained with the mammography unit offset 15° right and left. The coordinates of the lesion are entered into the computer from each stereo view. After preparing and locally anaesthetizing the skin of the breast at the calculated point of needle entry, a small stab wound is made and the biopsy needle mounted in a gun is advanced through the wound to the proper depth. "Prefire" stereoscopic views are taken to confirm that the biopsy needle is on target (Fig. 6.2B). One to five core needle biopsies are then taken, and a final image is procured prior to releasing the breast compression to confirm that the lesion demonstrates changes consistent with biopsy (Fig. 6.2C).

Like all needle biopsy techniques, the diagnostic accuracy of SCNB is subject to sampling error, which is comparable in magnitude to the probability of missing a mammographic lesion with NLBB.[10] Technical limitations of SCNB include difficulties in biopsying nonpalpable lesions situated close to the skin, in the immediate subareolar area or close to the chest wall. When a malignant diagnosis has been made, it is important that the skin entry site and parenchymal track of the core needle biopsy be excised en bloc with the definitive breast resection to prevent recurrence in the biopsy scar.[11] As with NLBB, benign results mandate close mammographic followup to apprehend the few neoplastic lesions which escape detection by this technique.

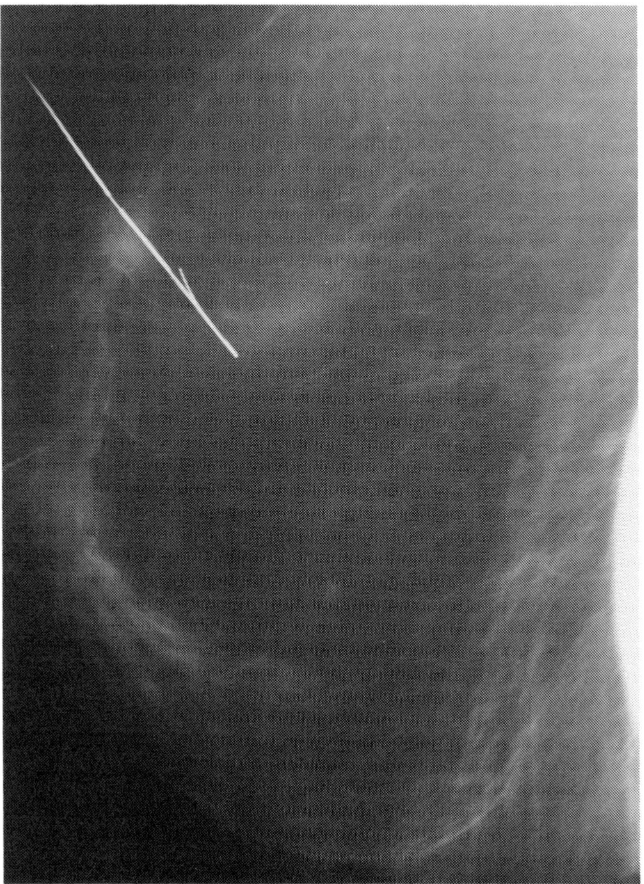

Fig. 6.1A

Fig. 6.1. Needle localization biopsy of the breast. In this patient, localization was performed using the mediolateral projection, the lesion of interest is a nonpalpable, spiculated soft tissue density in the superior portion of the breast. The Kopans wire is passed through the localizing needle into position and the hook deployed, thereby preventing dislodgement prior to or during the excisional biopsy procedure (A). After excision of the localized tissue, a mammogram of the specimen is taken with the wire in place to confirm that the abnormality of interest is within the excised tissue, and to assist the pathologist in identification of the lesion (B). The abnormality in this instance proved to be a carcinoma.

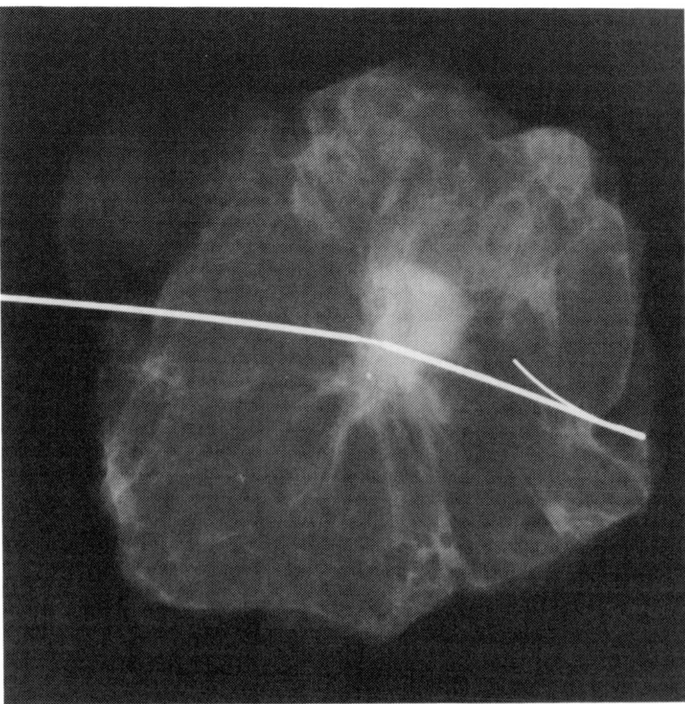

Fig. 6.1B

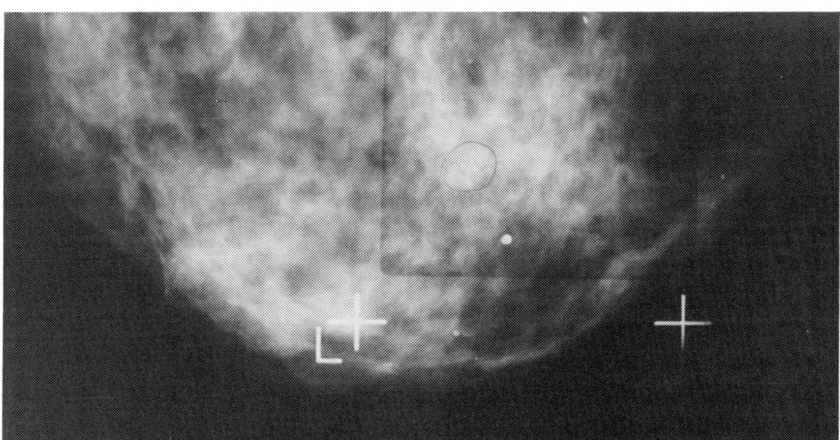

Fig. 6.2A

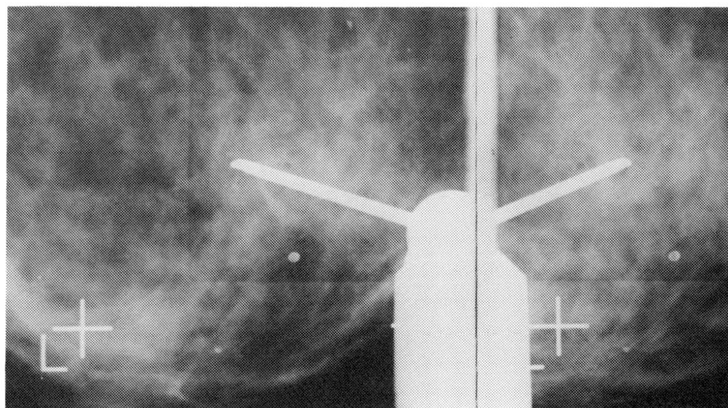

Fig. 6.2B

Fig. 6.2C

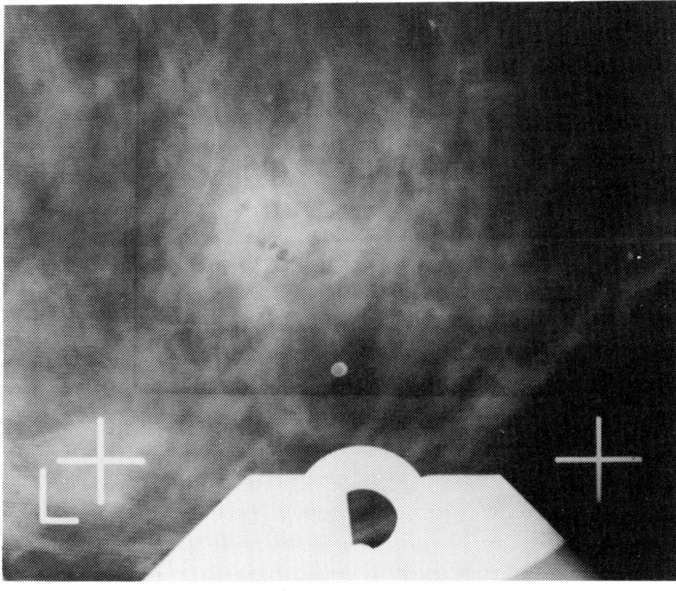

Fig. 6.2. Stereotactic core needle biopsy of the breast. With the patient suitably positioned (see text), the circled microcalcific soft tissue density is centered within the localizing window (A), stereoscopic views are taken and the coordinates of the lesion entered into the computer. The mounted core biopsy needle is then advanced through an appropriately placed cutaneous stab wound to the calculated depth, and "prefire" stereoscopic images are taken to confirm the accuracy of the localization (B). Following completion of the procedure, a final image is taken which in this case demonstrates air in the biopsy tracks, confirming that the needle transfixed the lesion and removed tissue from at least these three places (C). The final image more commonly shows increased soft tissue density within and around the abnormality due to hematoma. In this patient, the histopathological diagnosis proved to be fibrous mastopathy with microcalcifications.

DIAGNOSTIC CHALLENGES FOR THE PATHOLOGIST

Pathological nomenclature pertaining to benign, atypical and preinvasive breast disease is redundant and confusing, with many overlapping diagnostic terms. Independent review by several experienced pathologists of the same breast biopsy material occasionally yields diagnostic disparities ranging from benign proliferative changes to in situ and early invasive adenocarcinoma. Temple et al,[7] on careful pathological review of all in situ breast cancers in a Canadian provincial tumor registry, changed the diagnosis in 34% of cases. In addition, there were minor differences in diagnosis between the reviewing pathologists in 20% of cases, the most frequent points of disagreement relating to presence or absence of microinvasion and distinction of atypical hyperplasia from in situ carcinoma. This report underscores the diagnostic difficulties posed by many subclinical breast lesions. The diagnostic dilemma is most troubling for the treating physician and the patient; accurate distinction of true intraductal carcinoma, which should have essentially no potential for mortality, from ductal carcinoma in situ with microinvasion is of considerable importance in evaluating long term risks of recurrence and breast cancer mortality (see chapter 7).

The few patients with in situ breast cancer who subsequently develop axillary or distant breast cancer metastases would probably have been found to have early infiltrating disease in the breast if all submitted breast tissue had been meticulously sectioned and examined. This is impractical on a routine basis, but it is becoming standard practice to examine at least 15 to 30 tissue sections from in situ carcinomas to rule out infiltrating cancer. Larger lesions require especially careful examination; Lagios et al[12,13] reported that the risk of occult invasion in DCIS correlates with tumor size.

Misdiagnoses also result from overreading benign or atypical benign breast disease as in situ cancer, or in situ disease as invasive cancer. These misdiagnoses have been documented by the Surveillance Epidemiology and End Results (SEER) program,[14] the national breast cancer survey of the American College of Surgeons[15] and the Breast Cancer Detection Demonstration Projects (BCDDP).[16] On careful pathological re-evaluation of the submitted tissue sections from these three studies, over 50% of lesions originally identified as minimal breast cancer or microinvasive disease were found to be in situ cancer. Approximately 70% were DCIS and 30% LCIS.

CLINICAL SIGNIFICANCE OF DCIS

Ductal carcinoma in situ has a distinct profile and natural history, as summarized in several recent reviews.[17-19] These lesions parallel invasive breast cancer in terms of patient age at diagnosis. DCIS tends to be multifocal (within the same quadrant) or multicentric (involving more than one quadrant of the ipsilateral breast), and bilaterality is not infrequent. Axillary micrometastases are found 1% to 7% of the time, attesting to occult invasion of the breast stroma in at least a few patients diagnosed with pure DCIS. The 5- to 10-year risk of developing invasive breast cancer is estimated at 30% to 50%, and affects predominantly (but by no means exclusively) the ipsilateral breast in most series.

In the American College of Surgeons study, Rosner et al[15] reported a 50% to 60% incidence of residual in situ carcinoma in mastectomy specimens resected after breast biopsy. Synchronous invasive carcinoma was found in 5% to 50%, and metachronous invasive carcinomas occurred in 20% to 50% of patients followed for the long term.

Six series[20-25] have been published in which a total of 83 patients with DCIS were treated by excisional biopsy only. These suggest that there is a very high risk of recurrent in situ or metachronous invasive carcinoma at or near the biopsy site when DCIS has been incompletely excised (Table 6.1). At 4 to 10 years followup, the incidence of invasive cancer developing in the vicinity of the biopsy site was 25% to 75% (42% for all 83 patients). When DCIS is locally but completely excised with tumor-free margins, the incidence of invasive cancer at 3 to 7 years followup is 4% to 24% (Table 6.2). A

Table 6.1. The incidence of subequent invasive breast carcinoma following excisional biopsy only for ductal carcinoma in situ

Series	No. Patients	Histology	Subsequent Cancer	Mean Interval to Cancer (yrs)
Lewis[20]	8	Comedo	6 (75%)	4
Kraus[21]	4	Papillary/ Cribriform	2 (50%)	10
Farrow[22]	25	—	5 (25%)	8
Page[23]	25	Micropapillary/ Cribriform	7 (28%)	6
Betsill[24]	10	Papillary	7 (70%)	10
Haagensen[25]	11	Papillary	8 (73%)	10
TOTAL	**83**		**35 (42%)**	

Reproduced with permission from Ketcham AS, Moffat FL. Cancer 1990; 65:387-393.

Table 6.2. Treatment results with breast-conserving therapy for ductal carcinoma in situ of the breast

Series	No. Patients	Treatment	Recurrence Invasive	Noninvasive	Followup (yrs)
Temple[7]	17	BCS	6%	6%	>5
Lagios[12]	79	BCS	5%	1%	5
Lagios[13]	49	BCS	4%	2%	5
Ottesen[29]	112	BCS	4%	18%	4.5
Ciatto[30]	61	BCS	11%	—	>6
Schwartz[31]	70	BCS	4%	11%	4
Ringberg[32]	21	BCS	14%	—	7
Zafrani[26]	54	BCS + XRT	4%	2%	5
Fisher[27,28]	27	BCS + XRT	4%	4%	7
	21	BCS	24%	19%	7
Silverstein[30]	103	BCS + XRT	5%	5%	5
	26	BCS	4%	4%	1.5
Solin[34]	259	BCS + XRT	5%	5%	6.5
Cutuli[35]	36	BCS + XRT	6%	3%	4.5
Bornstein[36]	38	BCS+XRT	13%	8%	7

BCS breast-conserving surgery   XRT postoperative adjuvant breast radiotherapy

further 2% to 19% of patients developed more noninvasive carcinoma.

The incidence of multicentricity in intraductal cancers in total mastectomy specimens is reported as approximately 30%.[37-40] Multicentricity is much more frequent in palpable than in mammographically detected DCIS.[41] Holland et al[42] reported a high incidence of multifocality in a histopathological study of 32 intraductal lesions, and in 46% the true extent of tumor was underestimated by preoperative and specimen mammography. Lagios et al[9] reported multicentricity in 13 of 24 intraductal carcinomas of 25 mm size or larger, and in 4 of 29 smaller lesions. The potential therapeutic problem presented by multicentricity and multifocality has been a major focus of concern in the past. While recent prospective data[28,43] suggest that multicentricity in DCIS may not be clinically significant, this remains a point of legitimate concern at least for large palpable or diffuse multicentric DCIS.

RISK FACTORS FOR RECURRENCE

The risk for preinvasive or invasive recurrence is not uniform among patients with DCIS. Gump et al[41] compared grossly palpable with mammographically detected DCIS. They found that palpable DCIS had a much higher incidence of occult invasion and residual disease in the breast following excisional biopsy. Ottesen et al[29] reported that patients with clinically symptomatic DCIS experienced a 40% relapse rate following breast-conserving surgery, as compared to no recurrences among those whose intraductal cancers were found incidentally. They also reported an increased probability of recurrence when DCIS was macroscopic on gross inspection of the lumpectomy specimen, as compared to lesions detected only on microscopy. Occult invasion has also been related to tumor size by Lagios et al.[12,13]

DCIS has been classified into histological subtypes which correlate with biological behavior (Fig. 6.3). In situ comedocarcinoma or comedonecrosis associated with DCIS carries a greater long term risk for recurrence and is itself more apt to harbor microinvasion

or become invasive than papillary, cribriform or solid DCIS.[12,29,35,44,45] High histological grade also connotes aggressive behavior by itself[12,29] or when it occurs with comedonecrosis.[46] Lagios et al[12] reported that high tumor grade and aneuploidy correlate with comedocarcinoma and tumor necrosis, and are associated with a higher risk of local failure in the context of conservative surgery. These observations have been partly or wholly corroborated by others.[46,47]

Overexpression of the c-erbB-2 oncogene in DCIS correlates with a higher potential for invasiveness.[45-51] Transforming growth factor β_1, a regulatory protein important for cell growth, angiogenesis and possibly the invasive properties of tumor cells, was found in 12 of 18 invasive breast carcinomas and in 12 of 27 DCIS lesions (7 of 13 comedocarcinomas).[52] Oncogene products and growth factors could conceivably prove to be useful tools in discriminating between preinvasive cancers with low and high malignant potential.

THE AXILLA IN DCIS

Axillary metastases in the absence of demonstrable invasion in the primary tumor are uncommon in patients with DCIS. The incidence of axillary involvement associated with in situ cancer in the American College of Surgeons study was 1% to 4%.[15] Silverstein et al,[33,53] reported on 227 patients with DCIS without microinvasion, 163 of whom underwent axillary lymphadenectomy. They found no occult metastases in any case. Ashikari et

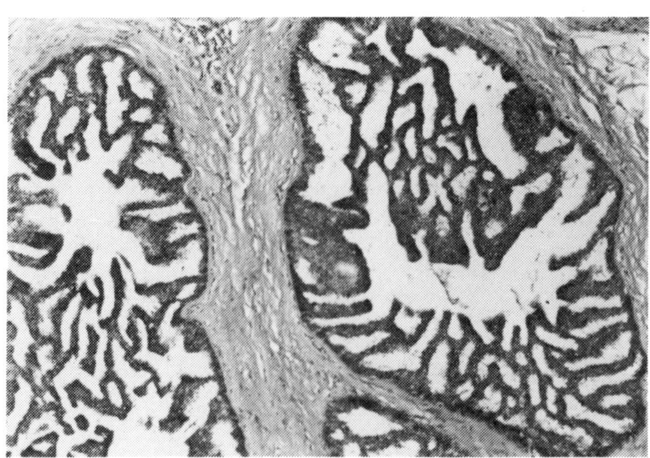

Fig. 6.3A. The histopathological subtypes of ductal carcinoma in situ. Papillary and micropapillary intraductal carcinoma (A) is characterized by small and large frond-like projections of neoplastic cells into the duct lumina, as seen in this 100x photomicrograph.

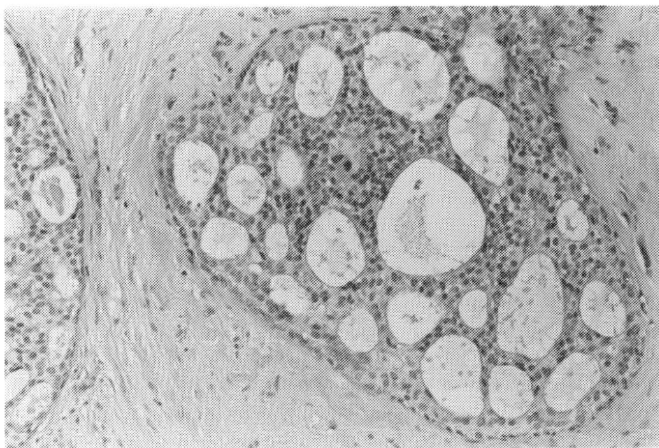

Fig. 6.3B. Cribriform DCIS, (B; 200x) is distinguished on cross-section by interlacing bands of tumors cells which seem to divide the duct lumen into multiple smaller passages.

Fig. 6.3C. Solid DCIS (C; 100x) is recognized by obliteration of the duct lumen by tumor cells without much necrosis.

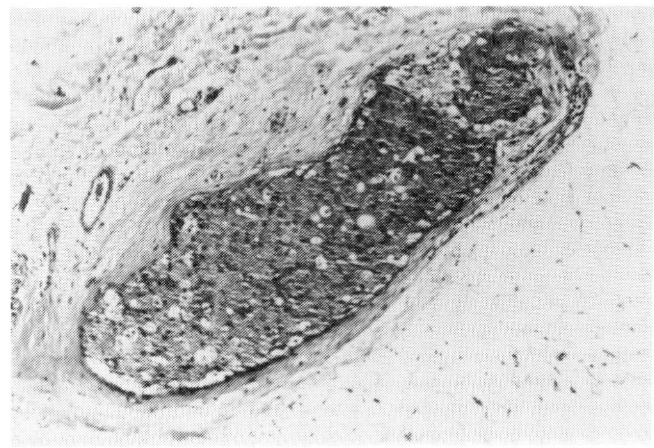

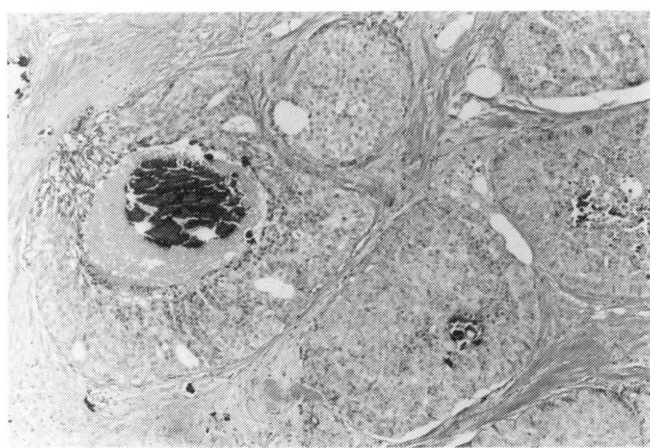

Fig. 6.3D. Intraductal comedocarcinoma (D; 100x), which tends to be a high grade lesion, characteristically fills the lumina with necrotic cells and debris as shown here. DCIS with comedonecrosis is associated with a higher risk of microinvasion, nodal metastases and disease-specific mortality than the other subtypes.

al[40] found only one patient with occult axillary disease in a series of 112 patients with DCIS, 109 of whom were subjected to axillary dissection as part of their treatment. Gump et al[41] reported 2 of 98 patients with palpable DCIS who had axillary metastases, as compared to no nodal involvement in any of their 24 patients with nonpalpable tumors. Of 87 patients with DCIS who underwent node sampling, Lagios et al[12] found axillary micrometastases in only two. Both had large lesions (68 and 160 mm) with focal microinvasion. Even with extensive DCIS, therefore, the case for axillary node biopsy or lymphadenectomy is less than compelling in the absence of unequivocal evidence of microinvasive disease or questionable clinical findings in the axilla.

The risk of metachronous contralateral breast cancer in patients with DCIS is substantial. Brown et al[39] reported contralateral invasive cancers in 4 of 40 patients treated and followed for DCIS. Webber et al[54] found four contralateral cancers in 116 patients with DCIS followed for an average of nine years. Two of 17 patients followed for a median time of 100 months by Gallagher et al[55] developed invasive cancers in the contralateral breast. Temple et al[7] reported the incidence of metachronous contralateral breast cancer to be very similar for DCIS and LCIS. Eight synchronous and 15 metachronous contralateral breast cancers were observed among 156 patients with DCIS reported by Ciatto et al.[30] The opposite breast is therefore a very significant concern in patients with a history of intraductal carcinoma.

PROGNOSTIC CONSIDERATIONS

The excellent prognosis of appropriately treated DCIS is compromised by the small likelihood of occult invasion and axillary micrometastases. Metachronous invasive breast cancers also contribute to disease-specific mortality. Invasive cancer following breast-conserving therapy for DCIS tends to arise in the same quadrant of the affected breast as the original in situ lesion.[17-22,23,24,27,28] Even with the most diligent clinical and mammographic followup, at least 20% to 30% of these new lesions have metastasized to the ipsilateral axilla by the time they are detected. Gallagher et al[55] reported three patients with invasive local recurrences in their series of 17 patients treated by breast-conserving surgery for DCIS. All three patients died of metastatic disease at a median interval of 131 months following recurrence.

Table 6.3. Results of the NSABP B-17 study at 43 months median followup comparison of BCS to BCS + XRT in patients with ductal carcinoma in situ[43]

	BCS		BCS + XRT	
Evaluable Patients	391		399	
Ipsilateral Breast Recurrences	64		28	
Noninvasive Recurrence	32	(10.4%)*	20	(7.5%)
Invasive Recurrence	32	(10.4%)	8	(2.9%)
Contralateral Breast Cancers	8		10	
Breast Cancer Deaths	1		2	

The difference in overall ipsilateral breast recurrences (noninvasive and invasive combined) was statistically significant (p = 0.001). The XRT-related reduction in noninvasive recurrences reached borderline significance (p = 0.055) while that related to invasive relapses was highly significant (p < 0.001).

*These percentages represent cumulative five-year recurrence rates.

BCS   breast-conserving surgery   XRT   postoperative adjuvant breast radiotherapy

Proponents of total mastectomy believe these factors strengthen the case for their preferred therapeutic approach to DCIS.

On the other hand, at least 50% of patients with DCIS never develop another breast neoplasm, suggesting that total mastectomy would be unnecessary in a majority of these women. It would be illogical to routinely recommend radical surgery for preinvasive cancer when early invasive disease can rationally be treated by local excision with or without radiotherapy.

TREATMENT OPTIONS

The incidence of invasive cancer or further in situ carcinoma in series in which DCIS was treated with wide local excision with or without postoperative breast radiation therapy ranges from 4% to 24% and 2% to 19% respectively (Table 6.2). The efficacy of radiotherapy in treatment of DCIS has been in doubt until very recently. Until the initial results of the NSABP B-17 trial[43] were reported, almost all data on radiation for intraductal carcinoma were from uncontrolled, usually retrospective studies. A short discussion of these follows.

In 14 patients followed for 7 to 45 months after local excision and radiation for DCIS, two recurrences were seen.[56] Recht et al[57] added 26 patients to this series, reporting satisfactory outcome with this regimen. Montague et al[58] documented 92% survival at 10 years followup in 54 nonrandomized patients treated by wide local excision and radiation. Solin et al,[34] reporting 10-year results in 259 patients from multiple North American and European centers, had 28 breast recurrences (16%), half of them invasive and half noninvasive. Four patients with breast recurrence went on to die of distant disease, and a further two patients died of metastases with no evidence of locoregional treatment failure. While these results seem promising, it is not possible to ascertain whether the use of ionizing radiations in these series resulted in improved treatment outcome as compared to surgery alone.

The NSABP B-06 trial included 76 patients in whom an initial diagnosis of microinvasive breast cancer was subsequently changed to DCIS by pathologists at NSABP headquarters.[27,28] Twenty-eight patients had been randomized to modified radical mastectomy, 27 to lumpectomy plus breast radiation, and 21 to lumpectomy without radiotherapy. At 87 months median followup, there were no differences in mortality or survival between treatment arms; one mastectomy and two lumpectomy patients had died of metastatic breast cancer. Local recurrence developed in two irradiated lumpectomy patients (7%) and 9 nonirradiated patients (43%). These data provided strongly suggestive evidence of the efficacy of adjuvant breast radiotherapy in the management of preinvasive breast cancer.

The prospective randomized NSABP B-17 trial[43] compared wide local excision to wide excision plus radiotherapy for in situ breast cancer. The EORTC has a similar trial in progress, the results of which have not been published as of this writing. Patients with completely excised DCIS (i.e., with histologically tumor-free margins) without evidence of invasive disease or axillary metastases were eligible for the B-17 trial. Patients with diffuse disease which could not be encompassed in a segmental mastectomy or other breast-conserving procedure were ineligible for this trial.

The results at a median followup time of 43 months are given in Table 6.3. While the proportion of ipsilateral breast recurrences outside the vicinity of the original lumpectomy (13.3%) is slightly higher than that observed in prospective randomized studies of breast conserving surgery for infiltrating cancer, the effect of radiotherapy on ipsilateral breast cancer recurrence, especially invasive recurrence, is highly significant. This study has provided the first incontrovertible evidence of the benefit of breast radiotherapy for intraductal carcinoma when used with breast-conserving surgery.

The NSABP has opened a second prospective randomized treatment trial for patients with DCIS. The B-24 study was designed to include patients with extensive DCIS, who would therefore have been ineligible for B-17. Extensive DCIS not amenable to complete removal by limited surgery still constitutes a large proportion of cases; these patients are usually offered mastectomy at the present time. In NSABP B-24, patients undergo breast-conserving surgery as in the earlier study; however, close or involved margins of resection or mammographic evidence of residual DCIS within the affected breast are not exclusion criteria as they were for NSABP B-17. All patients receive postoperative adjuvant breast radiotherapy, and are randomized to either tamoxifen or placebo treatment. The NSABP B-14 and other prospective clinical trials have demonstrated that tamoxifen reduces the incidence of contralateral breast cancer when used as adjuvant therapy for early invasive disease (see chapter 8). In addition, DCIS lesions are as frequently estrogen-receptor-rich as invasive carcinomas.[59] One of the biological questions being asked in B-24 is whether DCIS is in fact a reversible condition, and therefore preventable or controllable by the anti-initiator and anti-promotor activity of tamoxifen. The results of the NSABP B-24 study will shed new light on the therapeutic relevance of complete surgical extirpation to satisfactory long term treatment outcome for DCIS.

Total mastectomy has long been considered the treatment of choice for DCIS because of the high incidence of multicentricity and the tendency for recurrences to arise predominantly in the affected breast.

Silverstein et al[33] have recently reported a higher incidence of local recurrence with breast preserving therapy than with mastectomy despite a case selection policy in which only patients with smaller, more favorable DCIS lesions were treated conservatively. Total mastectomy does not eliminate the risk of recurrence or breast cancer mortality in patients with intraductal carcinoma (Table 6.4). A meta-analysis of treatment outcome on 895 patients from 12 series failed to show any survival differences between lumpectomy, lumpectomy plus radiation or total mastectomy, although lumpectomy alone was associated with a significantly higher local (breast) relapse rate.[63] So too, the American College of Surgeons retrospective survey showed no difference in five-year survival or recurrence rates between patients treated by conservative surgery or mastectomy for DCIS.[15] Nonetheless, in patients with diffuse, multicentric or large palpable intraductal carcinomas which are not amenable to breast preservation with clear surgical margins, total mastectomy with reconstruction is probably the most prudent approach outside of a clinical trial at the present time. If the B-24 trial demonstrates that tamoxifen effectively prevents DCIS recurrence even in the face of incomplete surgical excision, the role of total mastectomy in the management of intraductal carcinoma would likely be relegated to surgical salvage of local recurrence only.

Table 6.4. Recurrence and breast cancer mortality for ductal carcinoma in situ treated by total mastectomy or other radical operations

Series	No. Patients	Recurrences		Breast Cancer Mortalities
Lagios[13]	53	3	(5.7%)	1 (0.9%)
Rosner[15]	182	19	(10.4%)	– –
Fisher[27,28]	28	1	(3.6%)	1 (3.6%)
Ringberg[32]	111	1	(0.9%)	1 (0.9%)
Silverstein[33]	98	1	(1.0%)	0
Cutuli[35]	34	1	(3.0%)	1 (3.0%)
Ashikari[40]	112	1	(0.9%)	1 (0.9%)
Schuh[60]	51	1	(2.0%)	1 (2.0%)
von Rueden[61]	47	1	(2.1%)	0
Carter[62]	38	3	(7.9%)	3 (7.9%)
Total	**754**	**32**	**(4.2%)**	**9 (1.2%)**

In view of the controversies and uncertainties surrounding the treatment of DCIS, the patient herself must be carefully educated about what is known and not known about this entity. While many breast cancer patients will opt for breast-conserving therapy because of psychological, psychosexual and body image concerns, this perspective is not universally held. Some choose mastectomy and even bilateral ablative surgery because of reservations about retaining a "cancer-bearing" organ or fear of developing a new breast cancer in the future. Even when apprised of the unproven effectiveness of bilateral total mastectomy for breast cancer prophylaxis (see chapter 8), some of these patients will still request this operation. For them, peace of mind may best be served by the more radical approach to management, at least until such time as effective breast cancer chemoprevention is available. In the course of careful and thorough counselling, the patient must be given the time and latitude to arrive at an informed treatment decision which best fits her own temperament and personal philosophy.

TREATMENT DECISIONS

The NSABP B-17 results clearly demonstrate that wide local excision with postoperative adjuvant breast radiation is effective therapy for small to moderate-sized intraductal carcinomas completely excised in a breast-conserving operation. This approach is increasingly being employed by community surgeons as mammographic screening reveals DCIS lesions while they are still subclinical.[64] In the absence of unequivocal data concerning the efficacy of radiotherapy or tamoxifen when surgical margins are questionable or involved by DCIS, ipsilateral total mastectomy with or without breast reconstruction remains the most appropriate treatment for large or diffuse intraductal carcinomas outside of controlled clinical trials. Unless there is proven invasion or clinical suspicion of nodal spread, axillary lymphadenectomy is not indicated for DCIS.

In the American population, one in eight women will develop invasive breast carcinoma. DCIS connotes a risk for invasive cancer which is substantially greater than this, being of the same order of magnitude as the risk of contralateral carcinoma in breast cancer patients. Few surgical oncologists would advise (and even fewer breast cancer patients would accept) routine prophylactic contralateral mastectomy, and the case for routine total mastectomy for DCIS is just as precarious.

Subcutaneous mastectomy has been favored by some surgeons for in situ cancer because nipple preservation and infra-mammary incisions were felt to give an aesthetically superior result. Such cosmetic advantages as this operation may once have had are being overtaken by advances in post-mastectomy reconstructive surgical techniques. Moreover, as 5% to 15% of the breast parenchyma is left in situ when this procedure is performed,[65,66] there may be little if any abrogation of long term risk for breast cancer.[67-70] This operation should not be considered a satisfactory treatment alternative for neoplastic breast disease.

The patient with in situ breast cancer is entitled to full, unbiased disclosure of the facts and medical controversies surrounding treatment. All appropriate therapeutic options should be carefully outlined with attention to the advantages and drawbacks of each approach. It should not escape the American clinician's notice that several jurisdictions have passed statutes making such full disclosure mandatory for practitioners who treat breast disease. The patient must be apprised of the small but finite probability of breast cancer mortality attendant with either conservative or radical treatment, even in the face of compulsive clinical and mammographic followup. She should be made aware that this risk is not eliminated by removal of the affected breast and that mastectomy frequently amounts to over-treatment for her disease. The fully informed patient is usually willing to share the responsibility for her treatment and risk management if her philosophical predilections regarding cancer risk and cosmesis have been acknowledged and respected.

Whenever possible, patients should be encouraged to participate in prospective trials such as the EORTC study or the NSABP B-24 trial. More rapid accrual to such clinical trials is needed to answer questions about the biology and treatment of ductal carcinoma in situ.

REFERENCES

1. MacCarty WC. The histogenesis of cancer of the breast and its clinical significance. Surg Gynecol Obstet 1913; 17:441-446.
2. Broders AC. Carcinoma in situ contrasted with benign penetrating epithelium. J Amer Med Assoc 1932; 99:1670-1674.
3. Foote FW, Stewart FW. Lobular carcinoma in situ — a rare form of mammary cancer. Amer J Pathol 1941; 17:490-496.
4. Foote FW Jr., Stewart FW. Comparative studies of cancerous versus noncancerous breasts. Ann Surg 1945; 121:6-53.
5. Foote FW Jr., Stewart FW. A histologic classification of carcinoma of the breast. Surgery 1946; 19:74-99.
6. Page DL, Dupont WD, Rogers LW, et al. Atypical hyperplastic lesions of the female breast. Cancer 1985; 55:2698-2708.
7. Temple WJ, Jenkins M, Alexander F, et al. Natural history of in situ breast cancer in a defined population. Ann Surg 1989; 210:653-657.
8. Rusnak CH, Pengelly DB, Hosie RT, Rusnak CN. Preoperative needle localization to detect early breast cancer. Amer J Surg 1989; 157:505-507.
9. Elliott RL, Haynes AE, Bolin JA, Boagni EM, Head JF. Stereotaxic needle localization and biopsy of occult breast lesions: first years experience. Amer Surg 1992; 58: 126-131.
10. Parker SH, Lovin JD, Jobe WE, et al. Nonpalpable breast lesions: stereotactic automated large-core biopsies. Radiology 1991; 180:403-407.
11. Harter LP, Swengros-Curtis J, Ponto G, Craig PH. Malignant seeding of the needle track during stereotaxic core needle breast biopsy. Radiology 1992; 185:713-714.
12. Lagios MD, Margolin FR, Westdahl PR, et al. Mammographically detected duct carcinoma in situ. Frequency of local recurrence following tylectomy and prognostic effect of nuclear grade on local recurrence. Cancer 1989; 63:618-624.
13. Lagios MD, Westdahl PR, Margolin FR, et al. Duct carcinoma in situ. Relationship of noninvasive disease to the frequency of occult invasion, multicentricity, lymph node metastases and short-term treatment failures. Cancer 1982; 50:1309-1314.
14. Smart CR, Myers MH, Gloeckler LA. Implications from SEER data on breast cancer management. Cancer 1978; 41:787-789.
15. Rosner D, Bedwani RN, Vana J et al. Noninvasive breast carcinoma: results of a national survey by the American College of Surgeons. Ann Surg 1980; 192:139-147.
16. Beahrs OH, Shapiro S, Smart C. Report of the Working Group to review the National Cancer Institute — American Cancer Society Breast Cancer Detection Demonstration Projects. J Natl Cancer Inst 1979; 62: 643-709.
17. Ketcham AS, Moffat FL. Vexed surgeons, perplexed patients and breast cancers which may not be cancer. Cancer 1990; 65:387-393.
18. Frykberg ER, Bland KI. In situ breast carcinoma. Adv Surg 1993; 26:29-72.
19. Cady B. Duct carcinoma in situ. Surg Oncol Clin North Am 1993; 2:75-91.
20. Lewis D, Geschickter CF. Comedocarcinoma of the breast. Arch Surg 1938; 36:225-234.
21. Kraus FT, Neubecker RD. The differential diagnosis of papillary tumours of the breast. Cancer 1962; 15:444-455.
22. Farrow JH. Current concepts in the detection and treatment of the earliest of the early breast cancers. Cancer 1970; 25: 468-477.
23. Page DL, Dupont WD, Rogers LW, et al. Intraductal carcinoma of the breast: followup after biopsy only. Cancer 1982; 49: 751-758.
24. Betsill WL Jr., Rosen PP, Lieberman PH et al. Intraductal carcinoma. Long-term followup after treatment by biopsy alone. J Amer Med Assoc 1978; 239:1863-1867.
25. Haagensen CD. The papillary type of mammary carcinoma. In: Haagensen CD (Ed.). Diseases of the Breast (2nd ed.). Philadelphia, W.B. Saunders Co., 1971: 528-544.

26. Zafrani B, Fourquet A, Vilcoq JR et al. Conservative management of intraductal breast carcinoma with tumourectomy and radiation therapy. Cancer 1986; 57: 1299-1301.

27. Fisher ER, Sass R, Fisher B et al. Pathologic findings from the National Surgical Adjuvant Breast Project (Protocol 6). I. Intraductal carcinoma (DCIS). Cancer 1986; 57:197-208.

28. Fisher ER, Leeming R, Anderson S, et al. Conservative management of intraductal carcinoma (DCIS) of the breast. J Surg Oncol 1991; 47:139-147.

29. Ottesen GL, Graversen HP, Blichert-Toft M, et al. Ductal carcinoma in situ of the female breast. Short-term results of a prospective nationwide study. Amer J Surg Pathol 1992; 16:1183-1196.

30. Ciatto S, Grazzini G, Iossa A, et al. In situ ductal carcinoma of the breast — analysis of clinical presentation and outcome in 156 cases. Eur J Surg Oncol 1990; 16:220-224.

31. Schwartz GF, Finkel GC, Garcia JC, et al. Subclinical ductal carcinoma in situ of the breast. Treatment by local excision and surveillance alone. Cancer 1992; 70:2468-2474.

32. Ringberg A, Andersson I, Aspergren K, et al. Breast carcinoma in situ in 167 women — incidence, mode of presentation, therapy and followup. Eur J Surg Oncol 1991; 17:466-476.

33. Silverstein MJ, Cohlan BF, Gierson ED, et al. Duct carcinoma in situ: 227 cases without microinvasion. Eur J Cancer 1992; 28:630-634.

34. Solin LJ, Recht A, Fourquet A, et al. Ten-year results of breast-conserving surgery and definitive irradiation for intraductal carcinoma (ductal carcinoma in situ) of the breast. Cancer 1991; 68:2337-2344.

35. Cutuli B, Teissier E, Piat J-M, et al. Radical surgery and conservative treatment of ductal carcinoma in situ of the breast. Eur J Cancer 1992; 28:649-654.

36. Bornstein BA, Recht A, Connolly JL, et al. Results of treating ductal carcinoma in situ of the breast with conservative surgery and radiation therapy. Cancer 1991; 67:7-13.

37. Sunshine JA, Moseley HS, Fletcher WS, et al. Breast carcinoma in situ: a retrospective review of 112 cases with a minimum 10 year followup. Amer J Surg 1985; 150:44-52.

38. Peters TG, Donegan WL, Burg EA. Minimal breast cancer. A clinical appraisal. Ann Surg 1977; 106:703-710.

39. Brown PW, Silverman J, Owens E. Intraductal "non-infiltrating" carcinoma of the breast. Arch Surg 1976; 111:1063-1067.

40. Ashikari R, Hajdu SI, Robbins GF. Intraductal carcinoma of the breast (1960 - 1969). Cancer 1971; 28:1182-1187.

41. Gump FE, Jicha DL, Ozello L. Ductal carcinoma in situ (DCIS): a revised concept. Surgery 1987; 102:790-795.

42. Holland R, Veling SHJ, Mravunac M, et al. Histologic multifocality of Tis, T1-2 breast carcinomas. Implications for clinical trials of breast conserving surgery. Cancer 1985; 56:979-990.

43. Fisher B, Costantino J, Redmond C, et al. Lumpectomy compared with lumpectomy and radiation therapy for the treatment of intraductal breast cancer. New Engl J Med 1993; 328:1581-1586.

44. Gould EW, Morales AR. Incipient neoplasia of the breast. In: Albores- Saavedra J, Henson D (Eds.). Pathology of Incipient Neoplasia. Philadelphia, W.B.Saunders Co., 1986. Pp. 237-288.

45. Bellamy COC, McDonald C, Salter DM, et al. Noninvasive ductal carcinoma of the breast. The relevance of histologic categorization. Hum Pathol 1993; 24:16-23.

46. Solin LJ, Yeh I-T, Kurtz J, et al. Ductal carcinoma in situ (intraductal carcinoma) of the breast treated with breast-conserving surgery and definitive irradiation. Cancer 1993; 71:2532-2542.

47. Killeen JL, Namiki H. DNA analysis of ductal carcinoma in situ of the breast. A comparison with histological features. Cancer 1991; 68:2602-2607.

48. Lodato RF, Maguire HC, Greene MI, et al. Immunohistochemical evaluation of c-erbB-2 oncogene expression in ductal carcinoma in situ and atypical ductal hyperplasia of the breast. Mod Pathol 1990; 3:449-454.

49. Barnes DM, Meyer JS, Gonzalez JG, et al. Relationship between c-erbB-2 immunore-activity and thymidine labelling index in breast carcinoma in situ. Breast Cancer Treat Res 1991; 18:11-17.

50. Bartkova J, Barnes DM, Millis RR, et al. Immunohistochemical demonstration of c-erbB-2 protein in mammary ductal carcinoma in situ. Hum Pathol 1990; 21: 1164-1167.

51. Barnes DM, Bartkova J, Camplejohn RS, et al. Overexpression of the c-erbB-2 oncoprotein: why does this occur more frequently in ductal carcinoma in situ than in invasive mammary carcinoma and is this of prognostic significance? Eur J Cancer 1992; 28:644-648.

52. Walker RA, Dearing SJ. Transforming growth factor beta$_1$ in ductal carcinoma in situ and invasive carcinomas of the breast. Eur J Cancer 1992; 28:641-644.

53. Silverstein MJ, Rosser RJ, Gierson ED et al. Axillary lymph node dissection for intraductal breast carcinoma — is it indicated? Cancer 1987; 59:1819-1824.

54. Webber BL, Heise H, Neifeld JP, Costa J. Risk of subsequent contralateral breast carcinoma in a population of patients with in situ breast carcinoma. Cancer 1981; 47:2928-2932.

55. Gallagher WJ, Koerner FC, Wood WC. Treatment of intraductal carcinoma with limited surgery; long-term followup. J Clin Oncol 1989; 7:376-380.

56. Findlay P, Goodman R. Radiation therapy for treatment of intraductal carcinoma of the breast. Amer J Clin Oncol 1983; 6: 281-285.

57. Recht A, Danoff BS, Solin LJ et al. Intraductal carcinoma of the breast: results of treatment with excisional biopsy and irradiation. J Clin Oncol 1985; 3:1339-1343.

58. Montague ED. Conservation surgery and radiation therapy in the treatment of operable breast cancer. Cancer 1984; 53 (Suppl 3):700-704.

59. Chaudhuri B, Crist KA, Mucci S, et al. Distribution of estrogen receptor in ductal carcinoma in situ of the breast. Surgery 1993; 113:134-137.

60. Schuh ME, Nemoto T. Intraductal carcinoma. Analysis of presentation, pathologic findings and outcome. Ann Surg 1986; 121:1303-1307.

61. von Rueden DG, Wilson RE. Intraductal carcinoma of the breast. Surg Gynecol Obstet 1984; 158:105-111.

62. Carter D, Smith RL. Carcinoma in situ of the breast. Cancer 1977; 40:1189-1193.

63. Bradley SJ, Weaver DW, Bouwman DL. Alternatives in the surgical management of in situ breast cancer. A meta-analysis of outcome. Amer Surg 1990;56:428-432.

64. Coleman EA, Kessler LG, Wun L-M. Trends in the surgical management of ductal carcinoma in situ of the breast. Amer J Surg 1992; 164:74-76.

65. Goldman LD, Goldwyn RM. Some anatomical considerations of subcutaneous mastectomy. Plast Reconstr Surg 1973; 51: 501-505.

66. Georgiade N, Serafin D, Georgiade G, et al. Subcutaneous mastectomy: an evolution of concept and technique. Ann Plast Surg 1982; 8:8-19.

67. Pennisi VR, Capozzi A. The incidence of obscure carcinoma in subcutaneous mastectomy: results of a national survey. Plast Reconstr Surg 1975; 56:9-12.

68. Humphrey LJ. Subcutaneous mastectomy is not a prophylaxis against carcinoma of the breast: opinion or knowledge? Amer J Surg 1983; 145:311-312.

69. Jackson CF, Palmquist M, Swanson J, et al. The effectiveness of prophylactic subcutaneous mastectomy in Sprague-Dawley rats induced with 7,12-dimethyl-benzanthracene. Plast Reconstr Surg 1984; 73: 249-260.

70. Goodnight JE Jr., Quagliana JM, Morton DL. Failure of subcutaneous mastectomy to prevent the development of breast cancer. J Surg Oncol 1984; 26:198-201.

CHAPTER 7

Ductal Carcinoma In Situ with Microinvasion

The increased incidence of carcinoma in situ, carcinoma in situ with microinvasion and early infiltrating cancer in recent years is largely due to the widespread application of mammography. The prognostic implications of the mode of presentation of in situ and invasive cancer have been the subject of many studies. Breast neoplasms presenting clinically (palpable mass, nipple bleeding or discharge, Paget's disease) are further along in their natural history than those identified by mammography or as an incidental finding in breast biopsies performed for benign disease.[1-3] This is also true for breast cancers detected in asymptomatic women through clinical and mammographic screening.[1,4]

In 1971, Gallager and Martin[5] proposed the term "minimal breast cancer", encompassing DCIS, LCIS and infiltrating carcinomas of up to 0.5 cm in maximum diameter. Creation of this new category of breast cancer was prompted by the then-prevailing perception that because these lesions shared an indolent biological behavior and an excellent prognosis, they could be considered similar diseases for practical purposes. The ultrastructural anatomy of infiltration of malignant epithelial cells through the ductal basement membrane into the surrounding breast stroma was elucidated by Ozzello and Santipak.[6] This "microinvasive" state provided the unifying morphological link between in situ and early invasive breast cancer.

Several subsequent variations on the original definition of minimal breast cancer[7-12] have resulted in considerable confusion. As it has become clear that DCIS and LCIS do not always evolve into clinically important cancers, and that these entities differ from each other and from invasive cancer in important respects,[13] the term has become obsolete. Recognition that preclinical breast cancers have metastatic capability has focused attention on the risk of systemic tumor cell dissemination and resultant disease-specific mortality in cancers detected at the earliest stages of stromal infiltration.

As with minimal breast cancer, a single, universally accepted definition of "microinvasive" cancer does not exist. In general, the term is applied to lesions which are predominantly DCIS in which there is evidence of early tumor cell infiltration through the duct epithelial basal lamina into the surrounding breast stroma (Fig. 7.1). As progressively more stromal invasion is seen, the histological picture may ultimately merge with that of invasive carcinoma with an associated extensive intraductal component.

DCIS with microinvasion (DCISM) has been defined as one or more foci of invasion through the basement membrane in one or several ducts, the invasive disease comprising not more than 10% of the histological surface being examined.[1,3,14-20] Silverberg et al[12] examined risk of axillary metastases as a function of percent stromal invasion in patients with DCIS. Of 14 patients with less than 10% of histological sections showing stromal invasion, 2 of 11 undergoing axillary dissection had positive (3 or more) nodes as compared to 8 of 16 in whom stromal infiltration involved 10% to 49% of the histological surface area. Obviously, there is an element of subjectivity in such a classification; determination of whether there is less or more than 10% stromal invasion on the basis of histological sections is an imprecise discriminant for purposes of making treatment decisions.

Other authors prefer a more conservative definition of DCISM, this being evidence of tumor infiltration extending no further than 1 mm[21,22] or 2 mm[20,23] into the breast stroma. Still others have defined this entity simply as DCIS with evidence of early microscopic stromal infiltration.[2,24]

It has recently been suggested that dissection of the axillary lymphatics may not be indicated for DCISM.[19] Conceptually, this is very much in keeping with the trend away from mastectomy for infiltrating cancer, and from mastectomy and axillary lymph-adenectomy for DCIS. In essence, it is postulated that the risk of occult axillary metastases in patients with DCISM is closer to that of DCIS than true early invasive cancer, and therefore the potential morbidity of axillary lymphadenectomy is not justified. This hypothesis begs the question: if DCIS with focal invasion 1 to 2 mm into the surrounding stroma does not imply clinically important risk of axillary nodal involvement, at what point in the progression of parenchymal invasion by breast adenocarcinoma does the risk become significant?

CLINICOPATHOLOGICAL CORRELATES OF MICROINVASION IN DCIS

It stands to reason that DCISM should be a more advanced or intrinsically aggressive lesion than pure DCIS, and its clinical and histological characteristics tend to bear this out. DCISM presented more often with clinical findings (palpable mass, nipple discharge, Paget's disease) than DCIS in two series.[2,15] Moreover, DCISM was much less likely than intraductal carcinoma to be identified as an incidental finding in breast biopsies performed for benign pathology.[14,15] The incidence of microinvasion was found to be directly proportional to mammographic or pathological tumor size in several series.[21,23,25-27] All patients with DCISM in the series of Lagios et al[27] had lesions of over 4.5 cm in greatest dimension. Among the 208 patients reported by Silverstein et al,[21] only

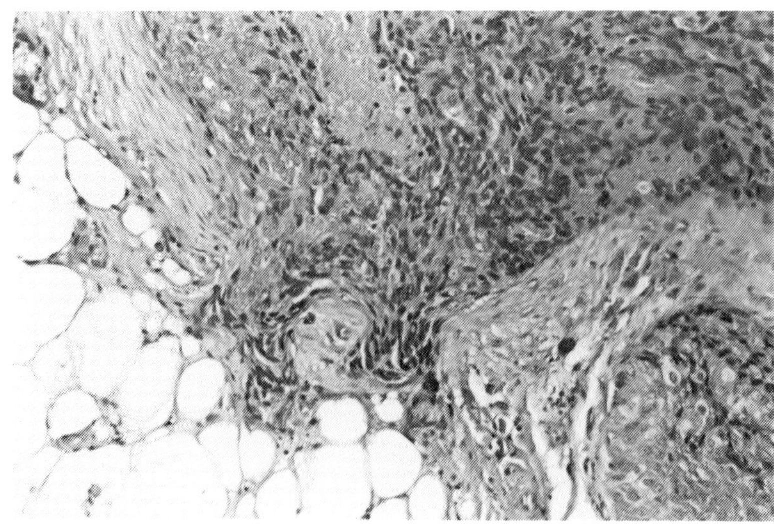

Fig. 7.1. Ductal carcinoma in situ with microinvasion. In this 100x photomicrograph, two longitudinally sectioned ducts containing DCIS are seen, one from the upper left and the other from the right. In the lower center, carcinoma is seen to infiltrate out of the duct into the surrounding stromal fat. This is an example of DCISM defined as invasion no more than 1 to 2 mm beyond the basement membrane.

5% of DCIS lesions 1 cm or less in diameter were DCISM, as compared to 19% of those over 1 cm; 24 of the 28 DCISM tumors in this series were larger than 1 cm, and 7 were over 5 cm in diameter.

Patchefsky et al[14] and Schwartz et al,[15] in examining the number of breast ducts containing DCIS in breast specimens, found that the incidence of microinvasion was directly proportional to the number of involved ducts. Significantly, however, there was no minimum number of involved ducts below which DCISM or multicentricity were never observed.

DCISM is multicentric more often than pure DCIS.[3,14,15,28] Residual cancer in postbiopsy mastectomy or lumpectomy specimens is found more frequently with DCISM than with simple DCIS.[3,14] While all of the foregoing observations suggest that microinvasion is most likely to be present in extensive intraductal carcinomas, it is nonetheless found with some frequency in even the smallest DCIS lesions.

DCISM is disproportionately associated with the comedocarcinoma histological subtype,[14,15,21,26,29-32] and tends to be poorly differentiated.[14,26,29]

THE RISK OF AXILLARY METASTASES AND MORTALITY IN DCISM

In light of the confusion surrounding the definition of DCISM, it is appropriate for comparative purposes to summarize the incidence of pathological node-positive disease among patients with early invasive breast cancers (Table 7.1). In particular, the American College of Surgeons[33] and the National

Table 7.1. Pathological node-positive axillae and disease-specific survival in early invasive ductal carcinoma

Series	Tumor Size (cm)	No. Patients	No. with AND	Confirmed pN+ Axillae		Followup	Five-Year Disease-free Survival pN–	pN+
Palpable and Nonpalpable Cancers								
Bedwani[33]	0.1 - 0.5	204	204	47	(23%)	5 yr	75.2%	51.1%
	0.6 - 1.0	1219	1219	255	(21%)	5 yr	69.5%	53.3%
Frazier[34]	0.1 - 0.5	21	?	2	(10%)	> 1 yr	—	—
Peters[35]	≤ 0.5	20	15	3	(20%)	—	—	—
Smart[36]	< 0.5	59	59	10	(17%)	—	—	—
	0.5 - 0.9	189	189	38	(20%)	—	—	—
								1-3 nodes / 4+nodes
Carter[37]	< 0.5	339	339	70	(21%)	5 yr	99%	95% / 59%
	0.5 - 0.9	996	996	205	(21%)	5 yr	98%	94% / 54%
Nonpalpable Cancers								
Schwartz[18]	≤ 0.5	7	7	4	(57%)	—	—	—
Margolis[22]	≤ 2.0	84	69	14	(20%)	—	—	64%
Ciatto[38]	≤ 0.9	38	34	1	(3%)	—	—	—
	1.0 - 1.9	78	69	9	(13%)	—	—	—
McKinney[39]	≤ 1.0	47	37	6	(16%)	—	—	—
Pagana[40]	≤ 1.0	49	31	4	(13%)	—	—	—
Wilhelm[41]	≤ 0.5	19	19	0	—	44 mo		67% }
	0.6-1.0	39	39	10	(26%)	44 mo	—	overall }
Tinnemans[42]	≤ 0.5	13	13	1	(8%)	68 mo	93%	80%
	0.6 - 1.0	24	24	3	(12%)	68 mo		— overall —
Reger[43]	≤ 0.5	34	≈34	1	(3%)	—	—	—
	0.6 - 1.0	144	≈144	14	(10%)	—	—	—
Silverstein[44]	≤ 0.5	96	96	3	(3%)	7 yrs		— 85% —
	0.6 - 1.0	156	156	27	(17%)	7 yrs		— 83% —

pN+ pathological node-positive   pN– pathological node-negative   AND axillary node dissection

Cancer Institute Surveillance, Epidemiology and End Results Program[36,37] data demonstrate quite clearly that the incidence of axillary metastases is approximately 20% among patients with invasive cancers of 5 mm or less in diameter. Moreover, patients with pathological node-positive cancers of 5 mm or less are much more likely to die of their disease than those with pathological node-negative tumors.

Published data on the incidence of pathological node-positive axillae and breast cancer mortality in DCISM are given in Tables 7.2 and 7.3. Like the early data on the natural history of untreated DCIS (Table 6.1), most of these series include few patients, and followup time is relatively short. The largest series[22] is that from the Connecticut Tumor Registry, in which DCISM was defined as focal microinvasion no more than 1 mm into the surrounding stroma. Axillary nodal metastases were found in 16% of patients in this study. The incidence of node-positive disease among these series ranges from 0 to 20%, with breast cancer mortality of 0 to 7%. These data do not allay concerns that the risk of pathological node-positive disease among patients with DCISM might approach that of patients with invasive cancers of 5 mm or less in size.

IS AXILLARY LYMPHADENECTOMY NECESSARY FOR DCISM?

There is no doubt about the prognostic and therapeutic significance of pathological node-positive breast cancer, irrespective of the size of the primary tumor. While chemotherapy is increasingly being recommended for axillary node-negative breast carcinoma, regimens for Stage I disease are less intensive (they often do not include alkylating agents such as cyclophosphamide) and of shorter duration than those employed for node-positive disease. Therefore, knowledge of axillary nodal status in individual patients with early breast cancer continues to be important. As long as axillary lymphadenectomy remains the only reliable means of determining nodal status in breast cancer patients, all those at significant risk for regional metastases should have an axillary staging procedure. As shown by the data in Table 7.1, up to 20% of the earliest infiltrating cancers have regional nodal disease at the time of diagnosis.

There is substantial confusion surrounding the definition of DCISM. It is not known whether there is a quantitative difference in risk of tumor dissemination between DCIS with one or more 1 mm foci of microscopic invasion and DCIS with microinvasion involving up to 10% of histological surface

Table 7.2. DCISM defined as focal microinvasion in predominantly DCIS lesions, with stromal invasion comprising 10% or less of the histological surface area being examined

Series	No. Patients	No. with AND	No. pN+		Followup	Breast Cancer Deaths
Palpable and Nonpalpable Lesions						
Rosner[3]	37	34	1	(3%)	48 mo	0
Silverberg[12]	14	11	2	(18%)	60 mo	0
Patchefsky[14]	16	16	3	(19%)	—	—
Wong[19]	41	33	0	(0%)	47 mo	0
Solin[20]	39	39	2	(5%)	55 mo	2 (5%)
Nonpalpable Lesions						
Schwartz[15]	13	13	1	(8%)	—	—
Schwartz[16]	25	25	0	(0%)	—	—
Schwartz[18]	10	10	0	(0%)	—	—

Table 7.3. DCISM defined by depth of microscopic stromal invasion in predominantly DCIS lesions

Series	Microscopic Stromal Invasion	Presentation	No. Patients	No. with AND	No. pN+	Followup	Breast Cancer Deaths
Schuh[2]	NOS	Palp + Nonpalp	30	30	6 (20%)	2-24 yrs	2 (6.6%)
Kinne[24]	NOS	Palp + Nonpalp	42	42	4 (10%)	11.5 yrs	3 (7.1%)
Silverstein[21]	≤ 1mm	Palp + Nonpalp	28	28	1 (3.6%)	45 mo	2 (7.1%)
Margolis[22]	≤ 1mm	Nonpalpable	137	137	22 (16%)	—	—
Radford[23]	≤ 2mm	Nonpalpable	27	27	3 (11%)	—	—

NOS not otherwise specified	Palp palpable	Nonpalp nonpalpable

area. The only available objective, clinically useful discriminant of metastatic potential in DCIS is the presence or absence of stromal invasion, irrespective of degree. The suggestion that minimal or microscopic invasion should connote little or no risk of tumor dissemination is somewhat reminiscent of the Halstedian concept of breast cancer biology.

The data on probability of axillary metastases in DCISM are sparse and followup is limited. However, the information summarized in Tables 7.2 and 7.3 does suggest that the risk of axillary nodal involvement in the presence of microinvasion may be in the range of 5% to 15%, higher than that associated with pure DCIS (see chapter 6). Rarely, even the apical axillary nodes have been involved.[42] More studies with longer followup are necessary before it can be determined with reasonable assurance that axillary surgical staging procedures can safely be avoided in patients with DCISM.

REFERENCES

1. Patchefsky AS, Shaber GS, Schwartz GF, et al. The pathology of breast cancer detected by mass population screening. Cancer 1977; 40:1659-1670.
2. Schuh ME, Nemoto T, Penetrante R, et al. Intraductal carcinoma. Analysis of presentation, pathologic findings, and outcome of disease. Arch Surg 1986; 121:1303-1307.
3. Rosner D, Lane WW, Penetrante R. Ductal carcinoma in situ with microinvasion. A curable entity using surgery alone without need for adjuvant therapy. Cancer 1991; 67:1498-1503.
4. Shapiro S, Venet W, Strax P, et al. Ten to fourteen year effect of screening on breast cancer mortality. J Natl Cancer Inst 1982; 69:349-355.
5. Gallager HS, Martin JE. An orientation to the concept of minimal breast cancer. Cancer 1971; 28:1505-1507.
6. Ozzello I, Sanpitak P. Epithelial-stromal junction of intraductal carcinoma of the breast. Cancer 1970; 26:1186-1198.
7. Ackerman LV, Katzenstein AL. The concept of minimal breast cancer and the pathologist's role in the diagnosis of "early carcinoma". Cancer 1977; 39:2755-2763.
8. Beahrs OH, Shapiro S, Smart C. Report of the Working Group to review the National Cancer Institute - American Cancer Society Breast Cancer Detection Demonstration Projects. J Natl Cancer Inst 1979; 62: 639-709.
9. Wanebo HJ, Huvos AG, Urban JA. Treatment of minimal breast cancer. Cancer 1974; 33:349-357.
10. Moskowitz M, Pemmaraju S, Filder JA, et al. On the diagnosis of minimal breast cancer in a screening population. Cancer 1976; 37:2543-2552.
11. Hayward J. Conservative surgery in the treatment of early breast cancer. Br J Surg 1974; 61:770-771.

12. Silverberg SG, Chitale AR. Assessment of significance of proportions of intraductal and infiltrating tumor growth in ductal carcinoma of the breast. Cancer 1973; 32: 830-837.

13. Wolmark N. Minimal breast cancer: advance or anachronism? Can J Surg 1985; 28: 252-255.

14. Patchefsky AS, Schwartz GF, Finklestein SD, et al. Heterogeneity of intraductal carcinoma of the breast. Cancer 1989; 63:731-741.

15. Schwartz GF, Patchefsky AS, Finklestein SD, et al. Nonpalpable in situ ductal carcinoma of the breast. Arch Surg 1989; 124:29-32.

16. Schwartz GF, Feig SA, Patchefsky AS. Significance and staging of nonpalpable carcinomas of the breast. Surg Gynecol Obstet 1988; 166:6-10.

17. Schwartz GF, Patchefsky AS, Feig SA, et al. Clinically occult breast cancer. Multicentricity and implications for treatment. Ann Surg 1980; 191:8-12.

18. Schwartz GF, Feig SA, Rosenberg AL, et al. Staging and treatment of clinically occult breast cancer. Cancer 1984; 53:1379-1384.

19. Wong JH, Kopald KH, Morton DL. The impact of microinvasion on axillary node metastases and survival in patients with intraductal breast cancer. Arch Surg 1990; 125:1296-1302.

20. Solin LJ, Fowble BL, Yeh I-T, et al. Microinvasive ductal carcinoma of the breast treated with breast-conserving surgery and definitive irradiation. Int J Radiat Oncol Biol Phys 1992; 23:961-968.

21. Silverstein MJ, Waisman JR, Gamagami P, et al. Intraductal carcinoma of the breast (208 cases). Clinical factors influencing treatment choice. Cancer 1990; 66:102-108.

22. Margolis DS, McMillen MA, Hashmi H, et al. Aggressive axillary evaluation and adjuvant therapy for nonpalpable carcinoma of the breast. Surg Gynecol Obstet 1992; 174:109-113.

23. Radford DM, Cromack DT, Troop BR, et al. Pathology and treatment of impalpable breast lesions. Amer J Surg 1992; 164:427-432.

24. Kinne DW, Petrek JA, Osborne MP, et al. Breast carcinoma in situ. Arch Surg 1989; 124:33-36.

25. Carter D, Smith RRL. Carcinoma in situ of the breast. Cancer 1977; 40:1189-1193.

26. Lagios MD, Westdahl PH, Margolin FR, et al. Duct carcinoma in situ. Relationship of noninvasive disease to the frequency of occult invasion, multicentricity, lymph node metastasis and short-term treatment failures. Cancer 1982; 50:1309-1314.

27. Lagios MD, Margolin FR, Westdahl PR, et al. Mammographically detected duct carcinoma in situ. Frequency of local recurrence following tylectomy and prognostic effect of nuclear grade on local recurrence. Cancer 1989; 63:618-624.

28. Schwartz GF, Patchefsky AS, Feig SA, et al. Clinically occult breast cancer. Multicentricity and implications for treatment. Ann Surg 1980; 191:8-12

29. Ottesen GL, Graversen HP, Blichert-Toft M, et al. Ductal carcinoma in situ of the female breast. Short-term results of a prospective nationwide study. Amer J Surg Pathol 1992; 16:1183-1196.

30. Cutuli B, Teissier E, Piat J-M, et al. Radical surgery and conservative treatment of ductal carcinoma in situ of the breast. Eur J Cancer 1992; 28:649-654.

31. Gould EW, Morales AR. Incipient neoplasia of the breast. In: Albores-Saavedra J, Henson D (Eds.). Pathology of Incipient Neoplasia. Philadelphia, W.B.Saunders Co., 1986: 237-288.

32. Bellamy COC, McDonald C, Salter DM, et al. Noninvasive ductal carcinoma of the breast. The relevance of histological categorization. Hum Pathol 1993; 24:16-23.

33. Bedwani R, Vana J, Rosner D, et al. Management and survival of female patients with "minimal" breast cancer: as observed in the long-term and short-term surveys of the American College of Surgeons. Cancer 1981; 47:2769-2778.

34. Frazier TG, Copeland EM, Gallager HS, et al. Prognosis and treatment in minimal breast cancer. Amer J Surg 1977; 133: 697-701.

35. Peters TG, Donegan WL, Burg EA. Minimal breast cancer: a clinical appraisal. Ann Surg 19 ; 186:704-710.

36. Smart CR, Myers MH, Gloeckler LA. Implications from SEER data on breast cancer management. Cancer 1978; 41:787-789.
37. Carter CL, Allen C, Henson DE. Relation of tumor size, lymph node status, and survival in 24,740 breast cancer cases. Cancer 1989; 63:181-187.
38. Ciatto S, Cecchini S, Iossa A, et al. Prognosis of nonpalpable infiltrating carcinoma of the breast. Surg Gynecol Obstet 1990; 170:61-64.
39. McKinney CD, Frierson HF, Fechner RE, et al. Pathologic findings in nonpalpable invasive breast cancer. Amer J Surg Pathol 1992; 16:33-36.
40. Pagana TJ, Lubbe WL, Schwartz SM, et al. A comparison of palpable and nonpalpable breast cancers. Arch Surg 1989; 124:26-28.
41. Wilhelm MC, Edge SB, Cole DD, et al. Nonpalpable invasive breast cancer. Ann Surg 1991; 213:600-605.
42. Tinnemans JGM, Wobbes T, Holland R, et al. Treatment and survival of female patients with nonpalpable breast carcinoma. Ann Surg 1989; 209:249-253.
43. Reger V, Beito G, Jolly PC. Factors affecting the incidence of lymph node metastases in small cancers of the breast. Amer J Surg 1989; 157:501-502.
44. Silverstein MJ, Gierson ED, Waisman JR, et al. Axillary lymph node dissection for T1a breast carcinoma. Is it indicated? Cancer 1994; 73:664-667.

CHAPTER 8

Lobular Carcinoma In Situ

Foote and Stewart[1] were the first to identify and characterize lobular carcinoma in situ (LCIS) with their classical description of its light microscopic appearance in 1941. They discovered the lesion in association with infiltrating carcinoma in 12 mastectomies, and as an isolated finding in a further 2 specimens.

LCIS has no clinical or gross pathological manifestations. The lesion arises from terminal ductal and lobular epithelium. Proliferation of cytologically abnormal cells produces distension of and luminal obliteration within the terminal duct-lobular complex without disrupting peripheral myoepithelial elements or lobular architecture (Fig. 8.1). The abnormal cells are large, round, well-differentiated and monotonously homogeneous in their appearance. There are no mitoses or necrosis.

Such cytological "indolence" can be a challenge for pathologists when the process involves only part of the terminal duct-lobule complex. Distinction of LCIS from atypical lobular hyperplasias (ALH) can be exceedingly difficult. As with DCIS, the diagnostic error rate for LCIS in the tumor registry study by Temple et al[2] was on the order of 30%. The most common discrepancies related to ALH and LCIS, but DCIS and invasive lobular carcinoma were occasionally miscoded as LCIS, and LCIS was misread in one instance as microinvasive ductal carcinoma.

Categorization of lobular disease of the breast is somewhat problematic. ALH and LCIS may represent two juxtaposed domains in the spectrum of lobular breast pathology, differing morphologically from one another only on quantitative grounds. A proliferation involving less than 50% of the acini in a breast lobule is considered ALH, whereas LCIS involves the majority of lobular acini.[3] The term lobular neoplasia, first coined by Haagensen[4] in 1978 in recognition that these entities do not manifest truly precancerous behavior, encompasses both ALH and LCIS.

LCIS has a much lower proliferative rate than invasive ductal carcinoma and comedo DCIS, as measured in thymidine labelling studies.[5] Overexpression of the c-erbB-2 oncogene is unusual, in contrast to DCIS.[6,7] Estrogen receptor positivity is much more prevalent for LCIS than intraductal comedocarcinoma.[8]

LCIS is usually an incidental finding in breast biopsy material or total mastectomy specimens. It is present in up to 10% of otherwise benign breast biopsies, and 30% to 40% of all in situ lobular lesions occur in association with invasive carcinoma. Although the incidence of diagnosis of LCIS has increased markedly since the advent of widespread mammographic surveillance, there are no radiographic characteristics which are pathognomonic or even suggestive of this lesion. Soft tissue or microcalcific mammographic changes mandating biopsy are rarely if ever found to correlate directly with the microscopic LCIS lesion; the LCIS is found in the grossly normal breast tissue resected with the mammographic abnormality (which itself is benign breast disease, DCIS or cancer).[9]

LCIS occurs mainly (80% to 90%) in premenopausal women and has a stronger proclivity for multicentric and bilateral distribution than DCIS. At the time of definitive treatment of LCIS by ipsilateral total mastectomy plus a contralateral breast operation (either biopsy or mastectomy), LCIS has been found in remote sites in the ipsilateral breast (relative to the diagnostic biopsy site) in 13% to 59% of cases,[10-13] and in the contralateral breast in 18% to 67%.[4,11-16] As with DCIS, the likelihood of axillary metastases in in situ lobular carcinoma is low, on the order of 1%.[17]

Since LCIS presents much less frequently in postmenopausal women, one must ask whether it regresses with age along with the lobular atrophy which follows menopause. Certainly, LCIS-related risk of invasive cancer does not decline with the passage of time. The risk is life-long; over 30% of metachronous breast cancers present more than two decades after the diagnosis of LCIS was made.[4,9,17]

THE CLINICAL SIGNIFICANCE OF LCIS

As LCIS is found mainly in premenopausal women, its peak incidence antedates that of infiltrating breast cancer by approximately 8 to 10 years. Moreover, the incidence of LCIS declines with age while that of invasive cancer increases. These observations would suggest that LCIS is a precursor of invasive breast cancer.

However, the preponderance of available evidence indicates that LCIS, unlike DCIS, is not a premalignant lesion in the classical sense. First, among patients with LCIS, most metachronous breast cancers are of ductal rather than lobular histology. Second, these breast cancers can arise with equal probability in any portion of either breast; unlike DCIS, the subsequent invasive cancers show no predilection for the particular site, quadrant or breast in which the in situ lobular carcinoma was initially found. Third, while the excess risk for metachronous cancer in DCIS patients is long-lived, it is especially protracted for LCIS. On balance, a much better case can be made for LCIS as an extraordinarily strong marker of risk for breast cancer.[18] LCIS may connote as much as a tenfold increase in risk for invasive breast cancer in affected individuals.[19]

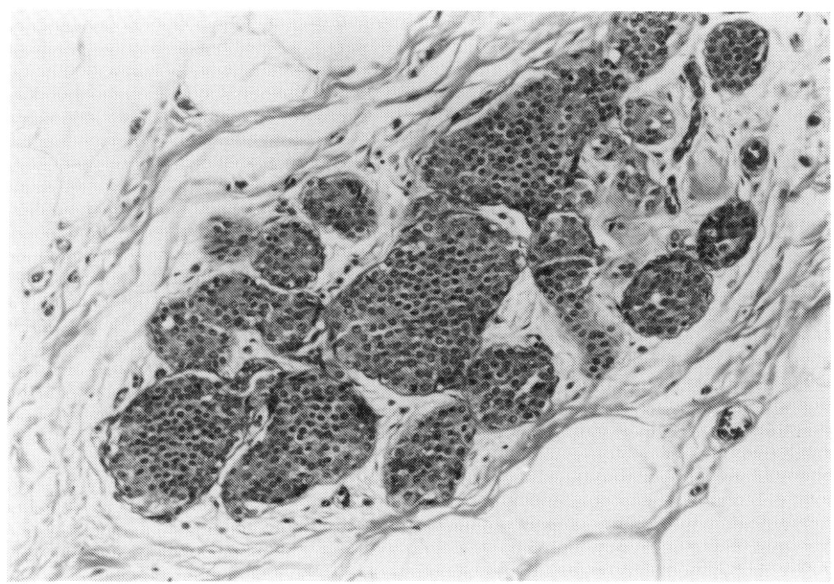

Fig. 8.1. Lobular carcinoma in situ. As shown in this 200x photomicrograph, the affected breast lobules are packed with abnormal lobular epithelial cells.

PROGNOSIS AND IMPLICATIONS FOR SURGICAL TREATMENT

The prognosis of LCIS is governed by its associated risk of metachronous invasive breast cancer. Page et al[3] have recently shown that the magnitude of this risk may be directly proportional to the extent of LCIS in the breast.

Published data regarding LCIS-related risk of ipsilateral and contralateral breast neoplasia and breast cancer mortality are given in Table 8.1. The proportion of patients developing second cancers over the periods of followup reported (6 to 24 years) ranged from 10% to 32%, the series of Sunshine et al[16] being the notable exception. Most of their 36 patients underwent bilateral mastectomy for LCIS; there was therefore little opportunity for metachronous cancers to develop. Invasive disease accounted for 53% of the second cancers in these twelve series. Most of the noninvasive second cancers were LCIS lesions. Second tumors were fairly evenly distributed over both ipsilateral and contralateral breasts; the relative paucity of metachronous ipsilateral and bilateral cancers in some series[11,12,20,21,24] is explained by the fact that significant numbers of these patients had undergone ipsilateral mastectomy as treatment for the original in situ lesion.

The most distressing consequence of LCIS is its associated breast cancer mortality, also summarized in Table 8.1. The overall incidence of breast cancer deaths for the twelve series was 4.5%. The only series reporting no breast cancer mortalities were the two[2,11] with the shortest followup and the smallest numbers of patients. The incidence of fatal outcome did not appear to be affected by treatment of the original LCIS lesion; patients in whom radical surgery was performed fared no better on the whole than those who were simply followed after the original diagnostic breast biopsy. A meta-analysis[25] of 780 LCIS patients from 13 series found no significant difference in breast cancer mortality between radical and conservative treatment for LCIS. Neither close surveillance, ipsilateral total mastectomy nor bilateral subcutaneous mastectomy[26-28] eliminates the possibility of metachronous invasive disease being discovered only after occult systemic dissemination has occurred. While LCIS may not fit the classical definition of a precancerous lesion, its significance is far from benign.

In an effort to obtain reliable prospective information on the natural history of LCIS, the NSABP B-17 trial registered 269 patients with in situ lobular carcinoma treated by local excision only. It is likely to be some time before data arising from this

Table 8.1. Treatment outcome in patients with lobular carcinoma in situ

Series	Followup (yrs)	No. Patients with 2nd Cancer/ Total No. Patients	No. Patients with Ipsilat. Cancer	No. Patients with Contralat. Cancer	No. Patients with Bilat. Cancer	Invas./Tot. 2nd Cancer*	Breast Cancer Deaths	
Temple[2]	6	4/30	3	1	0	2/4	0	
Page[3]	19	9/39	5	3	1	10/10	3	(7.7%)
Haagensen[4]	14	36/210	16	17	3	19/39	6	(2.9%)
Ringberg[11]	8	4/33	1	3	0	1/4	0	
Rosen[12]	14	29/101	10	19	0	7/29	4	(4%)
Andersen[13]	16	15/52	6	6	3	11/18	6	(11.5%)
Sunshine[16]	10+	0/36	0	0	0	1/1	1	(2.8%)
Rosen[17,22]	24	31/99	12	12	7	30/38	16	(16%)
Walt[20]	7.8	38/250	1	37	0	13/38	2	(0.8%)
Webber[21]	9	7/68	0	7	0	3/7	not given	
Hutter[23]	4-27	15/46	9	1	5	11/20	2	(4.1%)
Wheeler[24]	15.7	4/38	1	3	0	4/4	2	(5.7%)

* The total number of second cancers is the sum of the ipsilateral, the contralateral plus twice the number of bilateral cancers.

surveillance study are mature; there was no information about the LCIS patients in the initial report[29] of the B-17 study results.

LCIS-related risks of metachronous cancer and cancer mortality should theoretically be obviated by bilateral total mastectomy. However, this represents an extremely radical approach with potential benefit to only a small proportion of patients with LCIS. From this perspective, it is inconsistent to recommend radical surgery for preinvasive cancer when early invasive disease can rationally be treated with breast-conserving therapy.

That bilateral total mastectomy should provide definitive prophylaxis against breast cancer may seem intuitively obvious but remains unproven. Complete clearance of the anterior chest of breast tissue is highly dependent on surgical technique. Surgical excision of all breast parenchyma from the inferior mastectomy flap, the region of the axillary tail of Spence and lower axilla, and the anterior pectoralis major fascia is especially difficult. Breast parenchyma can be found within or even deep to the pectoralis fascia, on occasion.[30] While bilateral total mastectomy should provide the best assurance of breast cancer risk abrogation which surgery can offer, the experience with prophylactic oophorectomy in relatives of ovarian cancer patients should serve as an instructive caveat. Six of 324 such women who underwent prophylactic bilateral oophorectomy developed peritoneal carcinoma indistinguishable from ovarian adenocarcinoma after one to 27 years followup.[31] It cannot be assumed that bilateral total mastectomy completely eliminates the risk of future breast cancer.

BREAST CANCER CHEMOPREVENTION AND LCIS

There is convincing evidence from prospective randomized trials[32-36] and the recently published overview[37] of worldwide adjuvant therapy results that 2 to 5 years postoperative adjuvant tamoxifen for early invasive breast cancer significantly reduces the incidence of metachronous primary breast carcinoma.

The NSABP B-14 trial,[32,33] in which patients with node-negative estrogen receptor-positive breast cancer were randomized to tamoxifen or placebo, demonstrated an almost 50% reduction in metachronous contralateral breast cancers in the tamoxifen group; this effect was significant in both pre and postmenopausal patients. The B-14 trial also showed a significant reduction in ipsilateral breast relapses in tamoxifen-treated patients who had undergone breast-conserving surgery for the original tumor, and reduced incidence of regional nodal recurrence.

In the Stockholm Trial,[34] Stage I breast cancer patients were randomized to placebo or tamoxifen 40 mg/day for 2 to 5 years. At seven years median followup, second breast carcinomas had been found in 47 patients in the placebo group as compared to 29 tamoxifen-treated patients (p = 0.03). There was no difference between 2 and 5 years of tamoxifen therapy in terms of metachronous cancers. The Scottish Trial[35] and the Cancer Research Campaign Adjuvant Breast Trial[36] similarly show significant reductions in incidence of second primary breast carcinomas in patients randomized to tamoxifen 20 mg/day for 2 to 5 years following surgery for breast cancer.

The overview[37] of worldwide results with adjuvant tamoxifen in prospective randomized clinical trials found metachronous primary breast adenocarcinomas in 184 of 9,135 breast cancer patients (2.0%) on placebo as compared 122 of 9128 tamoxifen-treated patients (1.3%) (p < 0.00001). Reduction in second primary breast cancer incidence mediated by adjuvant tamoxifen has been an unexpected finding, but one which has been consistent across numerous controlled clinical trials employing many different experimental designs and therapeutic regimens.

The NSABP has recently opened the Breast Cancer Prevention Trial (BCPT), in which women at high risk for breast cancer are randomized to either placebo or tamoxifen 20 mg/day for a treatment period of at least five years. There are three categories of eligible participants, the first being women aged 60 years or older. Women aged 35 to 59 years whose risk of developing breast cancer is at least that of a 60-year-old, as determined by a risk estimate model developed by Gail et al,[38] are also eligible. The risk factors incorporated into the Gail model include number of first-degree relatives with breast cancer, nulliparity/age at first live birth, number of breast biopsies, histological diagnosis of atypical hyperplasia, and age of menarche.

Patients aged 35 years or older with a diagnosis of LCIS treated by local excision constitute the third category of eligible participants. LCIS is such a strong risk factor for breast carcinoma[19] that it is sufficient by itself as a criterion for inclusion in the BCPT for women aged 35 to 60 years. The BCPT has been accruing participants since May, 1992 from over 300 centers in the United States and Canada, and will include a total of 16,000 women. Approximately 4% of participants were women with LCIS at last report.[39]

TREATMENT DECISIONS

The conventional options include simple observation, wide local excision and ipsilateral or bilateral total mastectomy. Observation alone is certainly adequate for the incidentally discovered in situ lobular carcinoma which has been completely encompassed in the biopsy specimen. Radiotherapy has no role in the management of LCIS, in contradistinction to intraductal carcinoma. Similarly, in the absence of synchronous infiltrating carcinoma or clinical suspicion of nodal disease, axillary lymphadenectomy or biopsy is not indicated.

Of the surgical treatment options for LCIS, unilateral mastectomy has been the historical favorite. However, a unilateral ablative operation makes little sense for the bilateral risk posed by LCIS; the risk for future cancer is altered minimally or not at all. The only rational surgical options for LCIS are wide local excision with careful long-term surveillance, and bilateral total mastectomy. With the notable exception of those rare patients whose peace of mind is undermined by their "untreated" risk, patients and surgeons alike would concur that

bilateral mastectomy is an excessively radical approach to a locoregional risk which in at least 70% of cases never comes to fruition. Furthermore, the risk of metachronous cancer and mortality might not be completely eliminated by bilateral mastectomy, as noted above.

Whenever possible, patients with LCIS should participate in prospective studies such as the BCPT. The prospects for chemo-prevention of breast cancer in women with LCIS appear promising. Even if the BCPT ultimately demonstrates that tamoxifen is ineffective in this role, this trial will lead to a better understanding of breast cancer biology. As a general principle, local excision followed by participation in this or other prospective studies should be the "treatment option" of choice for patients with pure LCIS.

As with DCIS, the patient must be intimately involved in therapeutic decisions. If she is motivated, compliant and favorably disposed toward clinical trials, local excision and followup as a participant in the BCPT is optimal. Although the BCPT is a double-blind randomized study, the patient benefits from inclusion in this important clinical research effort. Participation in a clinical trial formalizes surveillance to a degree not usually attained in general clinical practice, and the patient may derive some abstract gratification from her involvement in a study which will answer important biological questions about breast cancer. It is important to emphasize to her that the BCPT is being conducted precisely because it is *not* known whether tamoxifen will prevent breast cancer in women with no previous history of infiltrating breast carcinoma; therefore, this drug cannot be properly prescribed for LCIS outside of a clinical trial.

For the reluctant patient or one who is ineligible for the BCPT because of a past history of another malignancy, deep venous thrombosis, depression, retinal disease, etc., wide local excision with careful followup is the most appropriate recommendation. For those whose temperament and sense of well-being are best served by ablative surgery, bilateral total mastectomy with or without breast reconstruction can be offered after thorough counselling about the controversies surrounding this option. Subcutaneous mastectomy should not be recommended to these high risk patients.

REFERENCES

1. Foote FW, Stewart FW. Lobular carcinoma in situ — a rare form of mammary cancer. Amer J Pathol 1941; 17:490-496.
2. Temple WJ, Jenkins M, Alexander F, et al. Natural history of in situ breast cancer in a defined population. Ann Surg 1989; 210:653-657.
3. Page DL, Kidd TE, Dupont WD, et al. Lobular neoplasia of the breast: higher risk for subsequent invasive cancer predicted by more extensive disease. Hum Pathol 1991; 22:1232-1239.
4. Haagensen CD, Lane N, Lattes R et al. Lobular neoplasia (so-called lobular carcinoma in situ) of the breast. Cancer 1978; 42:737-769.
5. Meyer JS. Cell kinetics of histological variants of in situ breast carcinoma. Breast Cancer Treat Res 1986; 7:171-180.
6. Ramachandra S, Machin L, Ashley S, et al. Immunohistochemical distribution of c-erbB-2 in in situ breast carcinoma: a detailed morphological analysis. J Pathol 1990; 161:7-14.
7. Porter PL, Garcia R, Mo R. c-erbB-2 oncogene protein in in situ and invasive lobular breast neoplasia. Cancer 1991; 68:331-334.
8. Bur ME, Zimarowski MJ, Schnitt SJ, et al. Estrogen receptor immunohistochemistry in carcinoma in situ of the breast. Cancer 1992; 69:1174-1181.
9. Kinne DW. Lobular carcinoma in situ. Surg Oncol Clin North Amer 1993; 2:65- 73.
10. Ashikari R, Huvos AG, Snyder RE. Prospective study of non-infiltrating carcinoma of the breast. Cancer 1977; 39:435-439.
11. Ringberg A, Andersson I, Aspegren K, et al. Breast carcinoma in situ in 167 women — incidence, mode of presentation, therapy and followup. Eur J Surg Oncol 1991; 17:466-476.
12. Rosen PP, Braun DW Jr., Lyngholm B, et al. Lobular carcinoma of the breast: preliminary results of treatment by ipsilateral mastectomy and contralateral breast biopsy. Cancer 1981; 47:813-819.
13. Andersen JA. Lobular carcinoma in situ. A long-term followup in 52 cases. Acta Path Microbiol Scand 1974; 82:519-533.
14. Newman W. In situ lobular carcinoma of the breast. Ann Surg 1963; 157:591- 599.
15. Urban JA. Bilateral breast cancer. Cancer 1969; 24:1310-1313.
16. Sunshine JA, Moseley HS, Fletcher WS, et al. Breast carcinoma in situ. A retrospective review of 112 cases with a minimum 10 year followup. Amer J Surg 1985; 150: 44-51.
17. Rosen PP, Braun DW Jr., Kinne DE. The clinical significance of preinvasive breast carcinoma. Cancer 1980; 46:919-925.
18. Ketcham AS, Moffat FL. Vexed surgeons, perplexed patients and breast cancers which may not be cancer. Cancer 1990; 65: 387-393.
19. Hutter RVP. Consensus meeting: Is "fibrocystic disease" of the breast precancerous? Arch Pathol Lab Med 1986; 110:171-173.
20. Walt AJ, Simon M, Swanson GM. The continuing dilemma of lobular carcinoma in situ. Arch Surg 1992; 127:904-909.
21. Webber BL, Heise H, Neifeld JP, Costa J. Risk of subsequent contralateral breast carcinoma in a population of patients with in situ breast carcinoma. Cancer 1981; 47:2928-2932.
22. Rosen PP, Lieberman PH, Braun DW Jr., et al. Lobular carcinoma in situ of the breast. Detailed analysis of 99 patients with average followup of 24 years. Amer J Surg Pathol 1978; 2:225-251.
23. Hutter RVP, Foote FW. Lobular carcinoma in situ: long term followup. Cancer 1969; 24:1080-1085.
24. Wheeler JE, Enterline HT, Roseman JM et al. Lobular carcinoma in situ of the breast: long term followup. Cancer 1974; 34: 554-569.

25. Bradley SJ, Weaver DW, Bouwman DL. Alternatives in the surgical management of in situ breast cancer. A meta-analysis of outcome. Amer Surg 1990; 56:428- 432.

26. Jackson CF, Palmquist M, Swanson J, et al. The effectiveness of prophylactic subcutaneous mastectomy in Sprague-Dawley rats induced with 7,12-dimethyl- benzanthracene. Plast Reconstr Surg 1984; 73: 249-260.

27. Pennisi VR, Capozzi A. The incidence of obscure carcinoma in subcutaneous mastectomy: results of a national survey. Plast Reconstr Surg 1975; 56:9-12.

28. Humphrey LJ. Subcutaneous mastectomy is not a prophylaxis against carcinoma of the breast: opinion or knowledge? Amer J Surg 1983; 145:311-312.

29. Fisher B, Costantino J, Redmond C, et al. Lumpectomy compared with lumpectomy and radiation therapy for the treatment of intraductal breast cancer. New Engl J Med 1993; 328:1581-1586.

30. Temple WJ, Lindsay RL, Magi E, et al. Technical considerations for prophylactic mastectomy in patients at high risk for breast cancer. Amer J Surg 1991; 161: 413-415.

31. Piver MS, Jishi MF, Tsukada Y. Primary peritoneal carcinoma after prophylactic oophorectomy in women with a family history of ovarian cancer. Cancer 1993; 71:2751-2755.

32. Fisher B, Costantino J, Redmond C, et al. A randomized clinical trial evaluating tamoxifen in the treatment of patients with node-negative breast cancer who have estrogen-receptor-positive tumors. New Engl J Med 1989; 320:479-484.

33. Fisher B, Costantino J, Wickerham L, et al. Adjuvant therapy for node- negative breast cancer: an update of NSABP findings. Proc Amer Soc Clin Oncol 1993; 12:69 (Abstr).

34. Rutqvist LE, Cedermark B, Glas U, et al. Contralateral primary tumors in breast cancer patients in a randomized trial of adjuvant tamoxifen therapy. J Natl Cancer Inst 1991; 83:1299-1306.

35. Breast Cancer Trials Committee, Scottish Cancer Trials Office. Adjuvant tamoxifen in the management of operable breast cancer. Lancet 1987; 2:171-175.

36. Abram WP, Baum M, Berstock DA, et al. Cyclophosphamide and tamoxifen as adjuvant therapies in the management of breast cancer. Preliminary analysis by the CRC Adjuvant Breast Trial Working Party. Br J Cancer 1988; 57:604-607.

37. Early Breast Cancer Trialists' Collaborative Group. Systemic treatment of early breast cancer by hormonal, cytotoxic, or immune therapy. 133 randomised trials involving 31,000 recurrences and 24,000 deaths among 75,000 women. Lancet 1992; 339: 1-15, 71-85.

38. Gail MH, Brinton LA, Byar DP, et al. Projecting individualized probabilities of developing breast cancer for white females who are being examined annually. J Natl Cancer Inst 1989; 81:1879-1885.

39. Redmond CK, Wickerham DL, Cronin W, et al. The NSABP Breast Cancer Prevention Trial (BCPT): a progress report. Proc Amer Soc Clin Oncol 1993; 12:69 (Abstr).

CHAPTER 9

THE CONTRALATERAL BREAST

The most significant risk factor for development of a new primary breast carcinoma is a previous history of breast cancer. The probability of a breast cancer patient harboring or developing a second primary breast adenocarcinoma has been calculated to be 437 per million women-years at risk[1] or 7.1 per year per thousand breast cancer patients. The latter estimate represents a cumulative incidence of about 0.7% to 1% per year,[2] essentially the same as that of second ipsilateral primary breast cancers following breast-conserving therapy (see chapter 3). The reported cumulative incidence of second primary breast cancer (both synchronous and metachronous) has ranged from 4.2% to 21%,[3-13] and most of these are metachronous (Table 9.1). Breast cancer patients are therefore roughly three times as likely to be faced with a second primary carcinoma as a woman in the general population is to develop her first breast tumor. In following patients who have undergone curative treatment for breast cancer, oncologists are acutely aware of the significant potential for further primary neoplasms to arise in either the conserved ipsilateral breast or the opposite breast.

The issue of bilaterality in breast cancer has been a focus of significant controversy in the literature. Much has been published on risk factors purported to connote especially high risk for second primary breast cancer, and the effect of a second primary cancer on overall breast cancer prognosis. The latter issue is of considerable interest from the standpoint of the management of the contralateral breast.

There has been a tendency in the literature to lump in situ and invasive breast cancer together when considering the risk of contralateral breast cancer and its management. While this may be appropriate to the extent that both infiltrating and in situ breast carcinoma imply heightened risk for second primary mammary cancer, it has added an element of confusion to discussions regarding the opposite breast.

The management options for the contralateral breast include close clinical and mammographic surveillance, selective or routine biopsy at the time of surgery for the first primary cancer, and prophylactic contralateral mastectomy. Decisions regarding the contralateral breast have often been based on evaluation of the perceived risk in the individual patient.

Table 9.1. Occurrence of bilateral breast cancer

Series	No. Patients	No. with Bilateral Cancer	No. with Synchronous Cancer	No. with Metachronous Cancer	Interval Between First and Second Cancers
Hermann[7]	418	31 (7.4%)	3 (0.7%)	28 (6.7%)	6.3 yrs
Al-Jurf[14]	5608	104 (1.8%)	26 (0.4%)	78 (1.4%)	123 mos
Burns[15]	1351	66 (4.9%)	3 (0.2%)	63 (4.7%)	10 yrs
Schell[16]	2231	106 (4.8%)	48 (2.2%)	58 (2.6%)	7 mos to 10 yrs
Bailey[17]	911	39 (4.3%)	17 (1.9%)	22 (2.4%)	68 mos
Buls[18]	–	76 –	21 –	55 –	≈5 yrs
Lewison[19]	490	42 (8.6%)	8 (1.6%)	34 (7.0%)	6 yrs
McLaughlin[20]	475	38 (8.0%)	– –	– –	≈5 yrs
Slack[21]	2734	52 (1.9%)	0 (0%)	52 (1.9%)	1-67 mos

Adapted and reproduced with permission from Wanebo HJ, et al. Ann Surg 1985; 201:667-677

RISK FACTORS FOR CONTRALATERAL BREAST NEOPLASIA IN BREAST CANCER PATIENTS

AGE

Breast cancer patients under the age of 45 years at the time of diagnosis may have an especially high risk of developing metachronous contralateral neoplasia.[1,2,4,5,22-25] In large population-based analyses from Connecticut, the United Kingdom and Denmark, patients in this age group were found to have a 4.9- to 5.5-fold greater chance of developing a contralateral breast cancer as compared to the risk for a first breast cancer in the general population. This compares to a relative risk of only 2.1 to 2.2 among breast cancer patients over the age of 55 at the time of diagnosis of their first primary.[1,22-24] Healey et al[13] also found younger breast cancer patients to be at significantly higher risk for a second primary mammary carcinoma.

However, Dawson et al[26] reported that early age was not a risk factor for bilaterality in their analysis.

PROGNOSIS AND STAGE OF THE FIRST PRIMARY BREAST CANCER

Published observations regarding the effect of the prognosis and stage of the first cancer on risk for contralateral breast carcinoma are contradictory. Certainly, it stands to reason that women whose first breast cancers have a favorable prognosis based on low stage, indolent histopathology or other factors might have a higher incidence of second primary breast cancer because their long survival eventuates in greater cumulative risk over time. This expectation has been confirmed in at least three studies.[2,10,27]

Patients with in situ breast neoplasia, either ductal or lobular, have a high risk of contralateral cancer as discussed below. This is undoubtedly in part because most of these women survive their disease and therefore remain at risk over a prolonged period of time. Simply because of the cumulative risk over time, the young patient with an excellent prognosis is likely to be at especially high risk for a second primary carcinoma.

The effect of stage of the first primary on risk for contralateral cancer is harder to gauge as published data are contradictory. Storm et al[23] and Hankey et al[24] concluded that more advanced stage in the first cancer connoted higher risk for synchronous or metachronous carcinoma in the contralateral breast. Robbins and Berg[2] and Hislop et al[5] found the opposite to be true, while Tulusan et al[4] and Lesser et al[28] found no relationship between risk for bilaterality and either the stage or nodal status of the first primary cancer.

FAMILY HISTORY OF BREAST CARCINOMA

As with stage and prognosis of the initial cancer, the effect of family history on risk for a second contralateral cancer is not clear cut. There have been a number of reports demonstrating excess risk for bilaterality in breast cancer patients with a positive family history,[3-5,23,29,30] but others have failed to demonstrate any association between familiality and bilaterality.[28,31,32] In particular, a population-based confirmatory study from Scandinavia[32] which was undertaken to corroborate Andersen's positive findings[30] failed to demonstrate any relationship between family history and contralateral breast cancer. Dawson et al[26] found no evidence for an association between bilaterality and familiality in their series.

HISTOPATHOLOGY OF THE FIRST CANCER

As already discussed in chapters 6 through 8, patients with ductal or lobular carcinoma in situ are at high risk for synchronous and metachronous second primary cancer, which can itself be either in situ or infiltrating.[3,4,9,33,34]

The histopathological subtype of the first primary cancer also has some bearing on the risk for bilateral breast carcinoma. Invasive lobular histology has been repeatedly shown to connote excess risk for contralateral cancer.[2,3,5,19,35] Patients with well-differentiated tubular adenocarcinomas have also been identified as being at higher than average risk for synchronous or metachronous bilateral breast cancer.[3,36]

Multicentricity in the original primary cancer, discussed in detail in chapter 2, also implies excess risk for carcinoma in the other breast.[2-5,28] Bilaterality and primary cancer multicentricity may simply be different manifestations of the same biological phenomenon.

Atypical fibrocystic disease in the vicinity of the first breast cancer was reported to marginally increase the excess risk for contralateral breast neoplasia in two studies.[3,5]

Tumor grade has been cited as a risk factor for contralateral breast cancer.[2,28] However, others have found no relationship in their analyses between this factor and the incidence of second breast cancer.[3-5]

SIZE OF THE FIRST PRIMARY CANCER

Reports from the National Surgical Adjuvant Breast Project (NSABP)[3,21] have identified patients with large first breast cancers as being at higher risk for carcinoma in the contralateral breast. However, an earlier study from Memorial Hospital, New York[2] had found that smaller tumors were associated with higher risk, while Tulusan et al[4] discerned no relationship between size of the first cancer and risk for a second.

THE USE OF RADIOTHERAPY IN TREATMENT OF THE FIRST CANCER

The available information on the effects of ipsilateral breast irradiation on the risk for contralateral breast cancer was reviewed in detail in chapter 3. Briefly, the opposite breast is unavoidably exposed to a low to moderate dose of ionizing radiations in the course of treatment of the cancer-bearing breast to a standard dose of 50 Gy. However, the radiation-related excess risk for contralateral breast cancer is slight, and may be of significance only in breast cancer patients with a long posttreatment life expectancy (i.e. young patients with an excellent outlook). Even in these individuals, the excess risk can only be demonstrated in studies of very large numbers of patients followed over long periods of time.

IS THERE AN IDENTIFIABLE SUBSET OF BREAST CANCER PATIENTS AT HIGH RISK FOR CONTRALATERAL BREAST CANCER?

From currently available information, it is impossible to discern a group of breast cancer patients which is at inordinately high risk for synchronous or metachronous cancer in the opposite breast. None of the variables associated with excess risk for contralateral breast cancer has a particularly strong influence; it is therefore not possible at the present time to target an identifiable high-risk subgroup for whom routine contralateral breast biopsy or prophylactic mastectomy could be undertaken with confidence that they would truly benefit from such aggressive intervention.

THE EFFECT OF A SECOND PRIMARY ON OVERALL LONG TERM BREAST CANCER PROGNOSIS

Unequivocal information on the prognostic impact of a second primary mammary carcinoma would be most helpful in determining the optimal management strategy for the contralateral breast at the time of diagnosis of the first breast cancer. However, once again the available data are mixed and leave considerable room for legitimate differences of opinion.

Robbins and Berg[2] reported 94 patients with bilateral breast cancer in whom the metachronous lesion was smaller than the initial primary and the incidence of axillary involvement was slightly lower for the second primary. The second cancer was found to have an adverse effect on overall breast cancer prognosis in this series. Fracchia et al[37] reported 403 breast cancer patients who developed a second cancer in the contralateral breast. Patients in whom both lesions were invasive carcinomas fared less well than patients with only unilateral breast cancer, and the prognosis was especially poor among those in whom both primaries had metastasized to the axilla. In essence, the probability of remaining disease-free with bilateral breast cancer was the product of the probability of remaining disease-free from each of the two carcinomas individually. Wanebo et al[6] also reported that the development of a second cancer in the contralateral breast was prejudicial to the long-term outlook; only 23% of patients with bilateral infiltrating carcinoma remained disease-free at 10 years. Healey et al[13] found that patients with metachronous contralateral breast cancer had a relative risk for distant metastasis of 2.

Robinson et al[12] studied 5,885 patients with synchronous and metachronous second breast cancers reported to the Surveillance, Epidemiology and End Results Program between 1973 and 1986. They found that the development of a second cancer was prejudicial to overall prognosis; for patients in whom both first and second cancers were pathologically node-negative, a small (5%) but significant reduction in survival at 13 years as compared to patients with only

unilateral breast cancer was found. For patients with node-positive first and second cancers, a 70% reduction in survival was identified.

However, two studies from the NSABP reached the opposite conclusion. Of 2,734 breast cancer patients entered into early NSABP prospective randomized trials, the long-term survival of 52 patients who developed a second cancer in the contralateral breast was no worse than that of patients with only unilateral disease.[21] Of the 1,578 patients in the NSABP B-04 study, 66 developed an additional contralateral cancer. At ten years followup, there was no evidence that the second cancer had adversely affected survival.[3] Graham et al[38] also reported that second primary breast cancer had no apparent effect on overall breast cancer prognosis.

Thus, it has not been clearly established that bilaterality adversely affects disease-free survival or disease-specific mortality. The data on prognostic influence of a second primary breast cancer do not clearly support routine contralateral breast biopsy (i.e. in the absence of questionable or suspicious findings) or prophylactic ablative surgery at the time of definitive management of the initial breast cancer.

ALTERNATIVES IN THE MANAGEMENT OF THE CONTRALATERAL BREAST

PROPHYLACTIC CONTRALATERAL TOTAL MASTECTOMY

While prophylactic contralateral mastectomy may apprehend all occult synchronous contralateral cancers at the earliest possible time, it has not been ascertained that total mastectomy is 100% prophylactic as regards metachronous breast cancer, as discussed in chapter 8. Moreover, in this day and age of breast conservation for biopsy-proven invasive breast cancer, recommendation of bilateral mastectomy on a routine basis is unsupportable; contralateral mastectomy in the absence of confirmed cancer or even suspicious clinical or mammographic findings cannot be justified in any but a very few, highly selected patients.[39] Prophylactic contralateral mastectomy is an extreme approach, and has adverse cosmetic and, in some women, psychological consequences.

In 91 breast cancer patients who underwent prophylactic removal of the opposite breast, Leis[40] found synchronous contralateral breast tumors in 16, 5 of which were invasive and 11 in situ carcinomas. At least 75 of the 91 mastectomies were therefore unnecessary in retrospect, and it is probable that at least some of the contralateral in situ cancers would never have come to light had mastectomy not been performed. There are no reliable criteria by which patients at high risk for synchronous or metachronous contralateral cancer can be identified and offered prophylactic mastectomy.[7]

Biopsy of the Contralateral Breast

The reported incidence of synchronous contralateral breast neoplasia is directly proportional to the effort expended to identify it. Contralateral breast biopsy on a routine, "blind" (i.e. in the absence of clinical or mammographic findings) basis will yield in situ and invasive breast cancers in only a small percentage of cases (Table 9.2). The yield from such routine (in essence random) biopsies increases with the volume of tissue excised and the diligence of the pathologist as evidenced by the number of tissue sections examined. However, most of these contralateral lesions are in situ carcinomas, at least some of which would not have become clinically problematic had mastectomy not been performed. Of 301 random biopsies performed by Urban et al,[8] neoplasms were identified in only 23; of these, only five were infiltrating carcinomas, for a yield of definite cancers of only 1.7%.

Pressman[47] reported a series of 247 contralateral breast biopsies performed in young high-risk patients, in which 32 neoplasms were found. Again, only four were invasive (1.6% of all biopsies). Similarly, Wanebo et al[6] discovered only three infiltrating carcinomas in 62 random contralateral breast biopsies. While the few patients in whom occult cancer is found by blind biopsy probably benefit from having their second cancers discovered while still preclinical, it is clear that the yield of such procedures is very low.

The in situ carcinomas which are found are problematic as it is not at all clear how these should be treated; this is especially true for lobular carcinoma in situ. In the present state of uncertainty, mastectomy is frequently recommended by the surgeon and accepted by the patient. Ablative cancer operations are therefore performed for lesions which in many cases were not fated to become true cancers.

Furthermore, in the absence of clinical or mammographic findings, contralateral breast biopsy will certainly miss a proportion of the synchronous in situ and invasive neoplasms. Smith et al,[46] in performing blind biopsies of the contralateral breast in 95 newly diagnosed breast cancer patients, found only two invasive cancers and three in situ lobular lesions, the latter of which of course

Table 9.2. Incidence of second cancers diagnosed by routine blind biopsy of the contralateral breast

Series	Incidence of Positive Biopsies
Urban[8,9]	12.5%
Fracchia[37]	12.7%
Leis[41]	7.6%
Fenig[42]	7.3%
Andersen[43]	5.9%
King[44]	4.5%
Martin[45]	2.0%
Smith[46]	5.5%

Modified and reproduced with permission from Wanebo HJ, et al. Ann Surg 1985; 201:667-677.

are not truly precancerous. Despite a negative blind biopsy, one additional patient developed a metachronous intraductal cancer in the opposite breast 19 months later. The net benefit of blind biopsy of the contralateral breast is likely very small, even in carefully selected patients.

Several advocates of routine blind contralateral breast biopsy recommend resecting up to 20% to 25% of the contralateral breast in doing these procedures.[6,8,9] The extent of these diagnostic operations exceeds that of segmental mastectomy for biopsy-proven infiltrating carcinoma in most surgeons' hands.

Most proponents of contralateral biopsy resect tissue from the upper outer quadrant and central regions of the breast. Some have also advocated biopsying the opposite breast at the mirror image location of the site of the known cancer in the ipsilateral breast.[6,8,9] Urban[9] explained this practice by stating that 40% of bilateral breast cancers are symmetrical in their presentation in the two breasts. However, a careful review of the literature has failed to reveal evidence to support this assertion.[48] Other than the statement that bilaterality in breast cancer implies symmetry, those who favor mirror image biopsy have apparently neither cited nor published any data which would suggest that the mirror image site in the contralateral breast is at uniquely high risk for occult neoplasia.

Clinical and mammographic evaluation of the opposite breast at the time of diagnosis of the first primary cancer may reveal questionable or suspicious changes for which biopsy is indicated. These directed biopsies are far more rewarding than those performed on a routine, blind basis in selected high-risk patients in whom there are no clinical or mammographic findings. In 28 newly diagnosed breast cancer patients with suspicious clinical or radiographic findings in the opposite breast, Urban et al[8] found 20 infiltrating and 2 in situ carcinomas. Pressman[47] found contralateral invasive lesions in all eleven patients with suspicious findings in the opposite breast.

CLINICAL AND MAMMOGRAPHIC SURVEILLANCE

Quarterly clinical assessments and annual mammography are the prevailing standard in North America and Europe for locoregional surveillance in breast cancer patients. After 3 to 5 years, the frequency of clinical followup is reduced unless disease recurrence supervenes.

Mahoney[49] reported 17 metachronous contralateral primaries in 466 patients over 10 years' followup. All lesions were palpable, and mammography was questionable or suspicious in seven cases. Urban et al[8] reporting in 1977 found that metachronous mammographically detected contralateral breast cancers were almost all invasive, and almost 50% had metastasized to the axilla by the time they were detected. Recent technical advances have made mammography the most sensitive noninvasive diagnostic modality for breast cancer. Mammography can often detect breast cancer at an early, preclinical stage.

Senofsky et al[50] compared the efficacy of clinical surveillance alone in 500 breast cancer patients before the advent of mammography to that of combined clinical and mammographic followup of 557 more recent patients. The 36 lesions found in the more recent group were diagnosed earlier during followup and were of lower stage than the 37 contralateral cancers found in the group followed by physical examination only. However, both clinical and mam-mographic surveillance were important; of the second cancers found in the more recent group, only 74% were seen on mammography.

Mellink et al[51] compared the efficacy of clinical examination alone as practised in Nijmegen, Holland to clinical examination plus mammography as used in Eindhoven for surveillance of the contralateral breast. Eight of 23 contralateral cancers diagnosed in Eindhoven were less than 1 cm in size when found, and 75% proved to be pathological node-negative. Of the 14 Nijmegen patients found to have metachronous contralateral breast cancer, only one had a tumor less than 1 cm, and eight (57%) were node-negative. They concluded that, while clinical examination can detect metachronous lesions in the opposite breast, the addition of mammography to the surveillance program results in earlier detection of new primary cancers.

Others have confirmed that clinical and mammographic surveillance are highly effective in detecting metachronous contralateral cancers at a very early stage.[52-54] Fisher et al[3] noted that contralateral tumors detected by mammography in NSABP B-04 patients were 1 cm smaller on average than the original primary cancers; moreover, there was no difference between the first and second cancers with respect to the incidence of axillary nodal metastases. They concluded that clinical and mammographic surveillance constitutes optimal management of the opposite breast in patients with early breast cancer. This was supported by their observation that second cancers had little prognostic significance, and by the fact that there is no clearly defined subset of patients which are at especially high risk for contralateral breast cancer.

CURRENT STATUS AND FUTURE PROSPECTS IN MANAGEMENT OF THE CONTRALATERAL BREAST

Of the three approaches to the problem of contralateral breast cancer outlined above, none is entirely satisfactory. As with breast cancer screening in normal women, close clinical and radiographic followup reduces but does not eliminate the risk of a second cancer escaping detection until metastatic spread has occurred. However, an aggressive approach which goes beyond clinically- or mammographically-directed biopsy of the opposite breast eventuates in unnecessary surgery being performed in a large majority of patients. As with so many other issues in breast cancer, the personal philosophy and temperament of a well informed patient and her physician or surgeon are very important factors in determining how best to address her risk for a second primary breast cancer.

As noted previously in this monograph, there is a very small number of women who, upon being diagnosed with breast cancer, will opt for bilateral mastectomies because of overwhelming anxiety about occult malignancy and the sense that both the cancer-bearing breast and the opposite gland represent a real hazard to their well-being. These sentiments can be refractory to the most diligent efforts on the part of surgical oncologists and general surgeons to persuade such patients that bilateral ablative surgery

constitutes overtreatment most of the time and may not completely eliminate the risk of metachronous breast carcinoma. For these few patients, prophylactic contralateral mastectomy is acceptable and even desirable from the standpoint of peace of mind. Advances in reconstructive surgery have made bilateral mastectomy a less mutilating undertaking than has been the case in years past.

For all other patients, a careful clinical examination and mammogram should be performed initially to rule out synchronous ipsilateral or contralateral breast cancer. Suspicious or questionable findings are biopsied, and treatment discussions and recommendations are predicated on the pathological findings.

While random biopsy of the contralateral breast has a low yield even in purportedly "high-risk" patients, it may be worthy of consideration in very young patients or those with multicentric or lobular carcinomas. When a second cancer is found in the opposite breast, bilateral breast cancer surgery is necessary, the extent of which is decided with the patient after careful discussion of all the issues, options and uncertainties in these difficult situations. For all others, quarterly posttreatment clinical examinations with annual mammography is most appropriate, with prompt biopsy of any interval changes.

Postoperative adjuvant tamoxifen significantly reduces the incidence of metachronous contralateral breast cancer, in addition to its many other beneficial effects in breast cancer patients.[55-58] This has been reviewed in previous chapters. Exploitation of such preventive measures should reduce the incidence of contralateral breast cancer, and thereby mitigate its impact on the psychological and disease-related morbidity, and perhaps the mortality, of breast cancer patients.

REFERENCES

1. Prior P, Waterhouse JAH. Incidence of bilateral tumors in a population-based series of breast cancer patients. I. Two approaches to an epidemiological analysis. Br J Cancer 1978; 37:620-634.

2. Robbins GF, Berg JW. Bilateral primary breast cancer. A prospective clinicopathological study. Cancer 1964; 17:1501-1527.

3. Fisher ER, Fisher B, Sass R, et al. Pathologic findings from the National Surgical Adjuvant Breast Project (Protocol No. 4). XI. Bilateral breast cancer. Cancer 1984; 54:3002-3011.

4. Tulusan AH, Ronay G, Egger H, Willgeroth F. A contribution to the natural history of breast cancer. V. Bilateral primary breast cancer: Incidence, risks, and diagnosis of simultaneous primary cancer in the opposite breast. Arch Gynecol 1985; 237:85-91.

5. Hislop TG, Elwood JM, Coldman AJ, et al. Second primary cancers of the breast: incidence and risk factors. Br J Cancer 1984; 49:79-85.

6. Wanebo HJ, Senofsky GM, Fechner RE, et al. Bilateral breast cancer. Risk reduction by contralateral biopsy. Ann Surg 1985;201:667-677.

7. Herrmann JB. Management of the contralateral breast after mastectomy for unilateral carcinoma. Surg Gynecol Obstet 1973; 136:777-779.

8. Urban JA, Papachristou D, Taylor J. Bilateral breast cancer. Biopsy of the opposite breast. Cancer 1977; 40:1968-1973.

9. Urban JA. Bilaterality of cancer of the breast. Biopsy of the opposite breast. Cancer 1967; 20:1867-1870.

10. Leis HP. Managing the remaining breast. Cancer 1980; 46:1026-1030.

11. McCredie JA, Inch WR, Alderson M. Consecutive primary carcinomas of the breast. Cancer 1975; 35:1472-1475.

12. Robinson E, Rennert G, Rennert HS, Neugut AI. Survival of first and second primary breast cancer. Cancer 1993; 71:172-176.

13. Healey EA, Cook EF, Orav EJ, et al. Contralateral breast cancer: clinical characteristics and impact on prognosis. J Clin Oncol 1993; 11:1545-1552.

14. Al-Jurf AS, Jochimsen PR, Urdaneta LF, Scott DH. Factors influencing survival in bilateral breast cancer. J Surg Oncol 1981; 16:343-348.

15. Burns PE, Dabbs K, May C, et al. Bilateral breast cancer in Northern Alberta: risk factors and survival patterns. Can Med Assoc J 1984; 130:881-886.

16. Schell SR, Montague ED, Spanos WJ Jr., et al. Bilateral breast cancer in patients with initial stage I and II disease. Cancer 1982; 50:1191-1194.

17. Bailey MJ, Royce C, Sloane JP, et al. Bilateral carcinoma of the breast. Br J Surg 1980; 67:514-516.

18. Buls JG, Bennett RC, Chan DPS. Bilateral carcinoma of the breast. Aust NZ J Surg 1976; 46:336-340.

19. Lewison EF, Neto AS. Bilateral breast cancer at the Johns Hopkins Hospital. Cancer 1977; 28:1297-1301.

20. McLaughlin CW Jr., Coe JD, Adwers JR. A thirty-year study of breast cancer in a consecutive series of private patients: is axillary nodal study a valuable index in prognosis? Amer J Surg 1978; 136:250-253.

21. Slack NH, Bross JD, Nemoto T, Fisher B. Experiences with bilateral primary carcinoma of the breast. Surg Gynecol Obstet 1973; 136:433-440.

22. Harvey EB, Brinton LA. Second cancer following cancer of the breast in Connecticut, 1935-1982. J Natl Cancer Inst Monogr 1985; 68:99-112

23. Storm HH, Jensen OM. Risk of contralateral breast cancer in Denmark 1943-1980. Br J Cancer 1986; 54:483-492.

24. Hankey BF, Curtis RE, Naughton MD Boice JD, Flannery JT. A retrospective cohort analysis of second breast cancer risk for primary breast cancer patients with an assessment of the effect of radiation therapy. J Natl Cancer Inst 1983; 70:797-804.

25. Chaudary MA, Millis RR, Hoskins EOL, et al. Bilateral primary breast cancer: a prospective study of disease incidence. Br J Surg 1984; 71:711-714.

26. Dawson PJ, Maloney T, Gimotty P, et al. Bilateral breast cancer: one disease or two? Breast Cancer Treat Rep 1991; 19:233-244.

27. Kilgore AR, Bell HG, Ahlquist RE. Cancer in the second breast. Amer J Surg 1956; 92:156-161.

28. Lesser ML, Rosen PP, Kinne DW Multicentricity and bilaterality in invasive breast carcinoma. Surgery 1982; 91: 234-240.

29. Chaudary MA, Millis RR, Bulbrook RD, Hayward JL. Family history and bilateral primary breast cancer. Breast Cancer Res Treat 1985; 5:201-205.

30. Anderson DE. Some characteristics of familial breast cancer. Cancer 1971; 28:1500-1504.

31. Wobbes T, van der Wiel WP, van der Sluis RF, Theeuves AGM. The effect of familiality on clinical presentation and survival in mammary carcinoma. Eur J Surg Oncol 1987; 13:119-121.

32. Adami H-O, Hansen J, Jung B, Rimsten A. Characteristics of familial breast cancer in Sweden: absence of relation to age and unilateral versus bilateral disease. Cancer 1981; 48:1688-1695.

33. Erdleich LS, Asal NR, Hoge AJ. Morphologic types of breast cancer: age, bilaterality and family history. South Med J 1980; 73:28-32.

34. Frykberg ER, Santiago F, Betsill WL, O'Brien PH. Lobular carcinoma in situ of the breast. Surg Gynecol Obstet 1987; 164:285-301.

35. Lewis TR, Casey J, Buerk CA, Cammack KV. Incidence of lobular carcinoma in bilateral breast cancer. Amer J Surg 1982; 144:635-638.

36. Lagios MD, Rose MR, Margolin FR. Tubular carcinoma of the breast. Amer J Clin Pathol 1980; 73:25-30.

37. Fracchia AA, Robinson DS, Legaspi A, et al. Survival in bilateral breast cancer. Cancer 1985; 55:1414-1421.

38. Graham MD, Yelland A, Peacock J, et al. Bilateral carcinoma of the breast. Eur J Surg Oncol 1993; 19:259-264.

39. Temple WJ, Lindsay RL, Magi E, Urbanski SJ. Technical considerations for prophylactic mastectomy in patients at high risk for breast cancer. Amer J Surg 1991; 161:413-415.

40. Leis HP. Selective, elective, prophylactic contralateral mastectomy. Cancer 1971; 28:956-961.

41. Leis HP. Bilateral breast cancer. Surg Clin North Am 1978; 58:833-841.

42. Fenig J, Arlen M, Livingston SF, Levowitz S. The potential for carcinoma existing synchronously on a microscopic level within the second breast. Surg Gynecol Obstet 1975; 141:394-396.

43. Andersen LI, Muchardt O. Simultaneous bilateral cancer of the breast - evaluation of the use of a contralateral biopsy. Acta Chir Scand 1980; 146:407-409.

44. King RE, Terz JJ, Lawrence W Jr. Experience with opposite breast biopsy in patients with operable breast cancer. Cancer 1976; 37:43-45.

45. Martin JK Jr., van Heerden JA, Gaffey TA. Synchronous and metachronous carcinoma of the breast. Surgery 1982; 91:12-16.

46. Smith BL, Bertagnolli M, Klein BB, et al. Evaluation of the contralateral breast. The role of biopsy at the time of treatment of primary breast cancer. Ann Surg 1992;216:17-21.

47. Pressman PI. Selective biopsy of the opposite breast. Cancer 1986; 57:577-580.

48. Moffat FL, Ketcham AS, Robinson DS, Legaspi A, Irani H. Breast cancer: management of the opposite breast. Oncology 1988; 2:25-30.

49. Mahoney L. Methods for detecting locally recurrent and contralateral second primary breast cancer. Can J Surg 1986; 29: 372-373.

50. Senofsky GM, Wanebo HJ, Wilhelm MC, et al. Has monitoring of the contralateral breast improved the prognosis in patients treated for primary breast cancer? Cancer 1986; 57:597-602.

51. Mellink WAM, Holland R, Hendriks JHCL, et al. The contribution of routine followup mammography to an early detection of asynchronous contralateral breast cancer. Cancer 1991; 67:1844-1848.

52. Missakian MM, Witten DM, Harrison EG. Mammography after mastectomy. Usefulness in search for recurrent carcinoma of the breast. J Amer Med Assoc 1965; 191:67-70.

53. Egan RL. Bilateral breast carcinomas. Role of mammography. Cancer 1976; 38:931-938.

54. Gutter Z. Cancer of the remaining breast: radiologic contribution to diagnosis. Can Med Assoc J 1976; 114:27-30.

55. Cuzick J, Baum M. Tamoxifen and contralateral breast cancer. Lancet 1985;2:282.

56. Fisher B, Costantino J, Wickerham L, et al. Adjuvant therapy for node-negative breast cancer: an update of NSABP findings. Proc Amer Soc Clin Oncol 1993; 12:69 (Abstr). breast cancer patients in a randomized trial of adjuvant tamoxifen therapy. J Natl Cancer Inst 1991; 83:1299-1306.

58. Early Breast Cancer Trialists' Collaborative Group. Systemic treatment of early breast cancer by hormonal, cytotoxic, or immune therapy. 133 randomized trials involving 31,000 recurrences and 24,000 deaths among 75,000 women. Lancet 1992; 339: 1-15, 71-85.

CHAPTER 10

THE TIMING OF BREAST CANCER SURGERY IN PREMENOPAUSAL PATIENTS

R ecent reports have suggested that the timing of surgical intervention relative to the menstrual cycle may affect breast cancer treatment outcome in premenopausal patients. This has aroused considerable interest and concern among the lay media and the public.

This hypothesis was first tested in humans in the late 1980s in a retrospective analysis of a small number of breast cancer patients.[1,2] The initial clinical study was itself prompted by the observation that survival and metastasis in an in vivo murine breast cancer model is profoundly influenced by the phase of the estrus cycle (the equivalent in rodents of the menstrual cycle) during which curative surgery is performed.[3] The premise that the timing of surgery with menstrual cycle phase might be important to long-term outcome had arisen from observations that natural killer lymphocyte activity and tumor hormone receptors vary significantly with the normal fluxes in circulating female hormones during the menstrual cycle.

Of all the risk factors (axillary nodal status, primary tumor size, tumor grade, hormone receptor status, etc.) established as prognostically important in breast cancer, none would be as readily susceptible to therapeutic manipulation as the timing of surgery; hence the high degree of interest in this possibility among the medical community, the press and the lay public. For this reason if for no other, a monograph focused on contemporary developments in locoregional breast cancer treatment would be incomplete without addressing this issue.

In this chapter, the experimental and clinical evidence supporting and discounting the hypothesis that timing of breast cancer surgery in premenopausal patients is important will be reviewed.

EFFECTS OF THE MENSTRUAL CYCLE ON IMMUNOLOGICAL FUNCTIONS AND TUMOR HORMONE RECEPTOR CONTENT

IMMUNOLOGICAL FUNCTIONS

Natural killer (NK) cells are a subpopulation of lymphocytes which, taken from unimmunized individuals, kill tumor cells in vitro independent of the presence of tumor-specific antibodies. In in vivo animal studies, the level of NK activity has been shown to influence both the growth rate of transplanted syngeneic tumors and the development of metastatic disease.[4,5] The antitumor cytotoxicity of NK cells is potentiated by interferons, and it is thought that NK cells are of pivotal importance in immune surveillance against spontaneously arising cancers in normal individuals.

White et al[6] assayed peripheral blood NK activity in 55 women undergoing breast biopsy and in 26 healthy controls. All blood samples were procured prior to biopsy. Of the 55 biopsied women, 23 proved to have benign lesions and the rest cancer. NK activity was significantly reduced in the cancer patients, but on further analysis this effect was found to be confined to those who were premenopausal. The NK activity of those with benign biopsies did not differ from that of the healthy controls for either pre or postmenopausal women. Among the cancer patients, there was no correlation between NK cytotoxicity and axillary node status, primary tumor size or tumor estrogen receptor status. In the premenopausal controls, those from whom the blood samples were procured in the first half of the menstrual cycle (the preovulatory, proliferative or follicular phase) showed significantly reduced NK cytotoxicity as compared to those who were assayed in the latter half (postovulatory, secretory or luteal phase).

Sulke et al[7] assayed peripheral blood NK cytotoxicity at three to four time points during the menstrual cycle in 18 healthy premenopausal women who were not taking oral contraceptives, 12 women taking the birth control pill and 7 normal males. In the 18 women not on oral contraceptives, NK activity decreased significantly following ovulation. In the women taking birth control medication and the men, NK activity did not fluctuate over time. No relationship was observed between NK cytotoxicity and circulating estradiol levels in any of the women.

In in vivo murine fibrosarcoma and melanoma models, Hanna et al[8] demonstrated that

β estradiol treatment decreased in vitro NK cytotoxicity by 50% to 85% and was associated with a significant increase in the number of pulmonary metastases for both tumor types. Thus, unopposed estrogen in this experimental setting was immunosuppressive and associated with greater tumor dissemination. This NK cell suppression was at odds with the findings of Sulke et al[7] which had suggested that the high-estrogen preovulatory phase of the human menstrual cycle was associated with greater NK cytotoxicity.

Thus, while these studies suggest that NK cytotoxicity fluctuates over the course of the menstrual cycle, their results otherwise tend to be contradictory. Whereas White et al[6] reported that NK cytotoxicity was low in the preovulatory phase, essentially the opposite was shown by Sulke et al.[7]

In studies of other aspects of immunity, it has been reported that phagocyte activity in female rodents varies directly with peripheral blood estrogen concentration.[9] In another study it was found that immune responsiveness to mitogens and sheep erythrocyte antigens followed a bimodal pattern, with one peak in proestrus and the other in metestrus (i.e. when circulating estrogen levels are at their highest and lowest, respectively).[10] A significant decrease in phagocytic function of mononuclear cells early in the preovulatory phase of the menstrual cycle has been reported in normal women.[11]

Tumor Hormone Receptors

Estrogen receptor-positive (ER+) breast cancer has a better long-term outlook than ER- disease. When it was first suggested that the timing of breast cancer surgery relative to the menstrual cycle might be prognostically significant, menstrual cycle-related variations in breast cancer ER status became of interest from the mechanistic standpoint.

Heise and Görlick[12] examined breast cancers from premenopausal and postmenopausal patients for estrogen receptor (ER) content. Of the 132 premenopausal patients, only 38% had ER positive (ER+) cancers as compared to 49% of cancers in the 167 postmenopausal patients. The mean ER content of tumors in the premenopausal group was significantly lower than that of cancers from postmenopausal patients (p < 0.001). Among the premenopausal group, the proportion of ER+ tumors and mean tumor ER content was highest when surgical excision was performed in the early proliferative phase of the menstrual cycle (1 to 7 days after the first day of the last menstrual period [LMP]) and lowest in early secretory phase (16 to 22 days after LMP), with a small increase in the proportion of ER+ tumors from days 23 through 28. This flux in proportion of ER+ tumors and tumor cell ER content was dramatic, exceeding the difference between pre and postmenopausal patients. While ER+ tumors have a better prognosis than ER- lesions, the authors were properly cautious about drawing conclusions regarding therapy. They attempted to explain these results by postulating that the increase in estradiol in early proliferative phase stimulates an increase in estrogen receptors, which by late proliferative phase are bound by circulating estradiol and translocate to the tumor cell nucleus. The progesterone surge which accompanies and follows ovulation stops further ER synthesis; therefore, as most of the preexisting ER have translocated to the nucleus, the proportion of ER+ breast cancers is lowest among those resected during the early secretory phase. At the end of the menstrual cycle, progesterone levels fall precipitously, ER translocation reverses direction and ER synthesis resumes under the recurring stimulus of estradiol, thereby repeating the cycle.

Axelrod et al[13] found only minor variation in breast cancer ER content related to the time of the menstrual cycle at which surgical excision was undertaken. Maximum ER positivity was seen in the early proliferative or preovulatory phase, although this difference was not significant. Progesterone receptor (PR) status did not vary with menstrual phase. While this study corroborated the finding of Heise and Görlick[12] that ER positivity is more frequent among breast cancers in postmenopausal patients, only minor fluctuations in ER content related to

the menstrual cycle were observed. These results were in agreement with those of Saez et al.[14]

Thus, as with the data on menstrual cycle-related variations in NK antitumor cytotoxicity, the findings regarding tumor ER content and timing of tumor excision are contradictory and inconclusive.

STUDIES SUGGESTING THAT TIMING OF BREAST CANCER SURGERY MAY HAVE PROGNOSTIC SIGNIFICANCE

MURINE STUDIES

Ratajczak et al[3] studied the effects of timing of surgery on breast cancer cure in an in vivo ER+ murine mammary carcinoma model. The murine fertility or estrus cycle, five days in length, was divided into two intervals for these experiments: proestrus/estrus, the periovulatory interval during which circulating estrogen levels and fertility are high and gonadotropin (FSH and LH) levels peak, and; metestrus/diestrus, characterized by low fertility and low plasma estrogen levels. Determination of estrus cycle phase was done by daily asessments of vaginal smear cytology for the duration of the experiment. Mammary carcinoma was inoculated into the hind extremity of test animals and allowed to grow for 14 to 17 days. The tumor-bearing extremity was then amputated at a time point consistent with either of the two estrus phases noted above, and the mice were followed for a further 28 days, sacrificed and the lungs examined grossly for metastatic tumor. The presence of pulmonary metastases was further sought in a bioassay in which lung tissue was transplanted into a second group of mice to determine whether viable tumor cells were present.

The time of tumor cell implantation relative to the estrus cycle, and the tumor size at amputation had no effect on numbers of metastases. Of the mice in which amputation was performed during proestrus/estrus, 27% had no pulmonary metastatic tumor as compared to 12% of those in which amputation was done during metestrus/diestrus (p = 0.035).

In a subsequent study, Hrushesky et al[15] reported that murine splenic NK cytotoxicity and interleukin-2 (IL-2) production varies rhythmically with the phases of the estrus cycle, and is highest during proestrus and estrus. NK cytotoxicity and IL-2 production therefore corresponded precisely with the optimal estrus cycle timing of breast cancer excision as determined by the murine pulmonary metastasis experiments. It was concluded that estrus cycle-related fluxes in NK cytotoxicity may be partially or wholly responsible for the estrus cycle-dependent differences in tumor metastasis.

Clinical Studies

Hrushesky et al[1] sought to put to a clinical test the hypothesis that timing of surgery is of prognostic importance in breast cancer. In a retrospective study of 41 premenopausal breast cancer patients for whom preoperative LMP data were available, clinical outcome was compared to the phase of the menstrual cycle which patients were in at the time of surgical intervention (excisional biopsy, lumpectomy, or mastectomy with or without axillary lymphadenectomy). These patients had been followed for 5 to 12 years from the time of the initial breast cancer surgery, and none had been on oral contraceptives. Patients were assigned to either of two menstrual groups based on time elapsed between first day of LMP and the date of surgery: days 7 to 20 (periovulatory or midcycle, 22 patients) and days 0 to 6 and 21 to 36 (perimenstrual, 19 patients). Breast cancer recurrence supervened in 8 of the 19 perimenstrual patients as compared to only 3 of the 22 periovulatory women (p < 0.05). The periovulatory group had a significantly longer disease-free survival (p = 0.016) and overall survival (p = 0.05). Multivariate analysis using the Cox proportional hazards model showed that timing of surgery was an independent predictor of disease-free survival and breast cancer mortality. When nodal status (a significant predictor of outcome in these patients) was controlled for, patients in whom surgery was performed in the perimenstrual phase of their menstrual cycle had a 4.5 times greater likelihood of treatment failure than the periovulatory group. Of the perimenstrual patients with ER- PR- cancers, 75% relapsed and 50% had died; none of the periovulatory patients with ER- PR- tumors had relapsed or succumbed to their disease at the time of publication.[2] While the authors noted the congruity between their murine experiments[2,3] and the clinical results in this analysis, they acknowledged that careful confirmation of these findings would be necessary before any recommendations could be made regarding changes in the practice of breast cancer surgery.

Three other positive clinical trials have been published, one from Guy's Hospital, London,[16,17] one from the Yorkshire Breast Cancer Group[18] and the other from Memorial Sloan-Kettering Cancer Center.[19,20] Badwe et al[16] reported a retrospective analysis of 249 breast cancer patients, testing the hypothesis that surgery during the time of unopposed estrogen stimulation leads to poorer survival. Based on the hormonal profile of the human menstrual cycle, they divided patients into those whose surgery was performed 3 to 12 days after the first day of the LMP (the unopposed estrogen group), and those who were operated upon 0 to 2 or 13 to 28 days after LMP (those with both circulating estrogen and progesterone at either low or high levels). The first group, consisting of 74 patients, had markedly reduced overall and disease-free survival as compared to the other patients (p < 0.001). Actuarial survival at 10 years for the first group was 54% and for the second, 84%. The differences in survival and recurrence were especially marked in node-positive patients. When the authors reanalyzed their data using the intervals studied by Hrushesky et al,[1,2] there was a 9% difference in survival at 10 years in favor of the perimenstrual patients; that is, the findings of this series were the opposite of those reported by Hrushesky et al. Nonetheless, they were sufficiently impressed by their observations that they changed their breast cancer practice so that premenopausal patients are operated upon at least 12 days after the onset of menses.

In a followup report analyzing 150 more recent patients, Badwe et al[17] confirmed their initial findings that patients operated upon during the unopposed estrogen phase (days 3 to 12 postLMP) fared worse in terms of disease-free survival.

Sainsbury et al[18] analyzed the prognostic influence of timing of first surgery (biopsy, lumpectomy or mastectomy) in 143 premenopausal patients in the Yorkshire Breast Cancer Group study for whom information on LMP was available. There was a difference of borderline significance (p = 0.06) in survival in favor of those undergoing surgery within 10 days of the onset of LMP, but no difference in disease-free survival. When reanalyzed using the intervals studied by Badwe et al,[16,17] the difference in overall survival for patients operated upon within 3 to 12 days of onset of LMP reached significance, but again, disease-free survival remained unaffected. The timing of surgery was not an independent predictor of survival or breast cancer dissemination on multivariate analysis.

Senie et al[19,20] reported 283 premenopausal breast cancer patients in whom the prognostic influence of the timing of surgery was compared in two ways; surgery performed during the periovulatory as compared to the perimenstrual phase as was done by Hrushesky et al,[1] and surgery performed during the follicular (days 0 to 14) as compared to the luteal phase (days 15 to 28). For the 27% of patients who underwent excisional biopsy prior to definitive breast cancer surgery, the date of the biopsy was used in this study. No differences were seen in the analysis of periovulatory versus perimenstrual surgical intervention. However, in the second analysis, disease-free survival was significantly lower in patients operated upon during the follicular phase. All of this difference was in patients with node-positive disease. ER and PR status was similar for both subsets of patients.

The studies in which timing of surgery was found to be a significant determinant in premenopausal patients do not concur on which phase of the menstrual cycle has the adverse effect on breast cancer recurrence and survival. Whereas Hrushesky et al[1] demonstrated a large survival difference in favor of

those operated upon in the periovulatory phase (days 7 to 20), Badwe et al[16,17] and Senie et al[19,20] failed to confirm this; rather, these studies showed that patients operated upon early in the menstrual cycle fared worse than those undergoing surgery later. However, there were important differences in the time intervals studied by these two groups of investigators. At best, the results from the Yorkshire Breast Cancer Group[18] provide marginal evidence of any effect of menstrual phase and timing of surgery on breast cancer outcome. Thus, like the studies on menstrual cycle-related fluxes in immunological function and tumor hormone receptor expression, there are very significant discrepancies between the studies which purport to show that timing of surgical intervention is a significant independent predictor of advers outcome in breast cancer patients.

STUDIES DEMONSTRATING NO PROGNOSTIC SIGNIFICANCE RELATED TO TIMING OF SURGERY AND THE MENSTRUAL CYCLE

A number of other retrospective studies showed statistically insignificant or no differences in premenopausal breast cancer outcome based on timing of surgery.[21-28] Donegan et al[23] failed to find an effect when either the time of initial biopsy or the time of definitive surgery was used in their analysis. Like the positive studies, the studies which showed no effect were also retrospective. The results and intervals tested for all studies, both positive and negative, are shown in Table 10.1.

The rather striking inconsistencies in the observations of the few positive studies and the fact that most failed to show any prognostic effect suggested the possibility that the positive analyses were spurious, chance findings. Moreover, the positive studies had tested different intervals of the menstrual cycle in their analyses. McGuire et al[29,30] noted that in statistically testing any hypothesis, there is a 5% chance of observing an effect when in fact none exists. With repeated testing when no effect exists, the probability of observing at least one positive result increases greatly (almost a 1 in 10 chance when

Table 10.1. Summary of the clinical studies of prognosis and the timing of breast cancer surgery with respect to onset of last menstrual period

Series	No. Patients	Menstrual Intervals Tested (days postLMP)			Significance
Hrushesky[1]	41	Days 7-20*	versus	Days 0-6 & 21-36	p < 0.05
Badwe[16]	249	Days 3-12	versus	Days 0-2 & 13-32*	p < 0.001
Badwe[17]	150	Days 3-12	versus	Days 0-2 & 13-33*	p < 0.001
Sainsbury[18]	143	Days 0-10*	versus	Days 11-32	p = 0.06
		Days 3-12*	versus	Days 0-2 & 13-32	p = 0.03
Senie[19,20]	283	Days 0-14	versus	Days 15-40*	p = 0.022
		Days 7-20	versus	Days 0-6 & 21-40	p = NS
Ville[21]	279	Days 7-20	versus	Days 0-6 & 21-36	p = NS
Gelber[22]	245	Days 7-20	versus	Days 0-6 & 21-36	p = NS
Donegan[23]	97	Days 7-20	versus	Days 0-6 & 21-36	p = NS
Powles[24]	81	Days 7-21	versus	Days 0-6 & 22-28	p = NS
Powles[25]	313	Days 3-12	versus	Days 0-2 & 13-32	p = NS
Gnant[26]	385	Days 3-12	versus	Days 0-2 & 13-32	p = NS
Marques[27]	235	Days 3-12	versus	Days 0-2 & 13-32	p = NS
Ville[28]	165	Perimenst vs follicular vs ovulatory vs luteal†			p = NS

* These intervals were associated with significantly better survival.
† Phase of menstrual cycle determined by peripheral blood hormone assays.

the experiment is performed just twice) but the probability of observing positive results consistently with repeated testing decreases dramatically to 100% • 0.05^X, where x is the number of times the experiment is repeated.

To test the possibility that all of the positive findings were the result of chance alone, McGuire et al[30] randomly assigned an integer from 1 to 28 to each of 675 breast cancer patients in the San Antonio Tumor Bank for whom treatment outcome was known. This integer represented a fictitious day of surgery related to the onset of LMP. They then analyzed the data repeatedly, comparing two 14-day menstrual cycle intervals or windows in each experiment. There were 14 possible pairs of 14-day windows, and it was found that windows starting on days 1, 2, 3, 4 and 14 yielded significant results with their random data. McGuire et al then repeated the experiment 100 times, each time randomly assigning new integers from 1 to 28 to the patients and testing each of the 14 possible pairs of 14-day windows with each new reassignment of integers. In 28 of the 100 trials, at least one 14-day pair of time intervals proved to yield significant differ-

ences in treatment outcome. However, there was no pattern to the significant windows; rather, they fit a random distribution (Fig. 10.1). The probability of finding a spuriously significant result was calculated as 30%.

CONCLUSION

The lack of congruity among the positive retrospective analyses suggests strongly that these are in fact chance findings. This is further supported by the numerous negative studies and by McGuire's elegant demonstration of the effects of chance on repeated analysis of random data. Definitive investigation of this question would require a multicenter prospective study in which patients are randomly allocated to surgical treatment at two or more points in the menstrual cycle. Because of the marked variability in the length of the menstrual cycle, assays of peripheral blood sex hormone levels would be required to verify the point of the cycle at which each patient was operated upon. Ideally, immunological parameters would be assessed as well. All of this presumes, of course, that there is a consensus on which intervals from LMP to surgery and what immune functions should be tested.

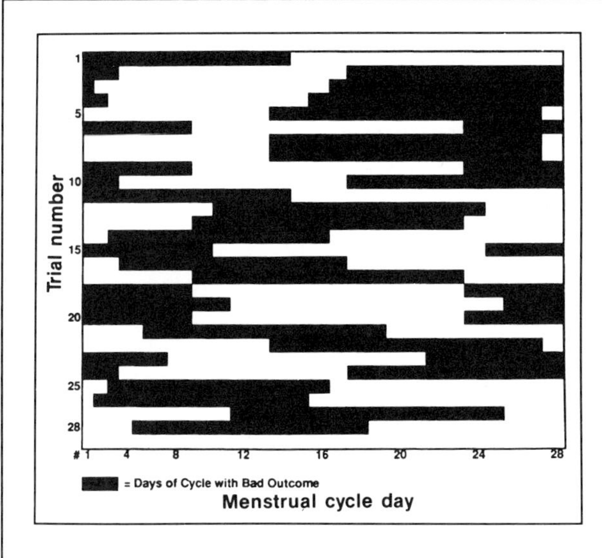

Fig. 10.1. A graphic summary of the 28 statistically significant 14-day pairs of menstrual cycle windows found in the 100 trials of the random experiment performed by McGuire et al.[30] Reproduced from McGuire WL, et al. J Natl Cancer Inst 1992; 48:346-348.

Such a consensus would be difficult to reach, given the conflicts among the currently available studies. It is doubtful whether such a prospective study will be performed, and a few investigators have questioned whether such an effort would be warranted, given the inconsistencies and the large number of negative studies.[23,26] Certainly, there is no justification at present for altering surgical scheduling practices for premenopausal breast cancer patients.

References

1. Hrushesky WJM, Bluming AZ, Gruber SA, Sothern RB. Menstrual influence on surgical cure of breast cancer. Lancet 1989; 2:949-952.

2. Bluming A, Hrushesky WJM. The effect of surgical timing within the fertility cycle on breast cancer outcome. Ann NY Acad Sci 1991; 618:277-291.

3. Ratajczak HV, Sothern RB, Hrushesky WJM. Estrous influence on surgical cure of a mouse breast cancer. J Exp Med 1988; 168:73-83.

4. Kiessling R, Wigzell H. An analysis of the murine NK cell as to structure, function and biological relevance. Immunol Rev 1979; 44:165-208.

5. Hanna N. Expression of metastatic potential of tumor cells in young nude mice is correlated with low levels of natural killer activity. Int J Cancer 1980; 26:675-680.

6. White D, Jones DB, Cooke T, Kirkham N. Natural killer (NK) activity in peripheral blood lymphocytes of patients with benign and malignant breast disease. Br J Cancer 1982; 46:611-616.

7. Sulke AN, Jones DB, Wood PJ. Variation in natural killer activity in peripheral blood during the menstrual cycle. Br Med J 1985; 290:884-886.

8. Hanna N, Schneider M. Enhancement of tumor metastasis and suppression of natural killer cell activity by ß-estradiol treatment. J Immunol 1982; 130:974-980.

9. Nicol T, Vernon-Roberts B. The influence of estrus cycle, pregnancy and ovariectomy on RES activity. J Reticuloendothel Soc 1965; 2:15-29.

10. Krzych U, Strausser HR, Bressler JP, et al. Quantitative differences in immune responses during the various stages of the estrous cycle in female BALB/c mice. J Immunol 1978; 121:1603-1605.

11. Stratton JA, Miller RD, Kent DR, et al. Depressed mononuclear cell phagocytic activity associated with menstruation. J Clin Lab Immunol 1984; 15:127-131.

12. Heise E, Görlick M. Estradiol receptor in human breast cancers throughout the menstrual cycle. Oncology 1982; 39:340-344.

13. Axelrod DM, Menendez-Botet CJ, Kinne DW, Osborne MP. Levels of estrogen and progesterone receptor proteins in patients with breast cancer during various phases of the menses. Cancer Invest 1988; 6:7-14.

14. Saez S, Martin PM, Chouvet CD. Estradiol and progesterone receptor levels in human breast adenocarcinoma in relation to plasma estrogen and progesterone levels. Cancer Res 1978; 38:3468-3473.

15. Hrushesky WJM, Gruber SA, Sothern RB, et al. Natural killer cell activity: age, estrus- and circadian-stage dependence and inverse correlation with metastatic potential. J Natl Cancer Inst 1988; 80: 1232-1237.

16. Badwe RA, Gregory WM, Chaudary MA, et al. Timimg of surgery during menstrual cycle and survival of premenopausal women with operable breast cancer. Lancet 1991; 337:1261-1264.

17. Badwe RA, Richards MA, Fentiman IS, et al. Surgical procedures, menstrual cycle phase, and prognosis in operable breast cancer. Lancet 1991; 338:815-816.

18. Sainsbury R, Jones M, Parker D, Hall R, Close H. Timing of surgery for breast cancer and the menstrual cycle. Lancet 1991; 338:392.

19. Senie RT, Rosen PP, Rhodes P, et al. Prognosis of primary breast cancer patients in relation to time of diagnostic surgeryduring the menstrual cycle. Breast Cancer Res Treat 1990; 16:146 (Abstr).

20. Senie RT, Rosen PP, Rhodes P, Lesser ML. Timing of breast cancer excision during the menstrual cycle influences duration of disease-free survival. Ann Intern Med 1991; 115:337-342.

21. Ville Y, Lasry S, Spyratos F, Hacène K, Brunet M. Menstrual status and breast cancer surgery. Breast Cancer Res Treat 1990; 16:119.

22. Gelber RD, Goldhirsch A. Menstrual effect on surgical cure of breast cancer. Lancet 1989; 2:1344.

23. Donegan WL, Shah D. Prognosis of patients with breast cancer related to the timing of operation. Arch Surg 1993; 128:309-311.

24. Powles TJ, Jones AL, Ashley S, Tidy A. Menstrual effect on surgical cure of breast cancer. Lancet 1989; 2:1343-1344.

25. Powles TJ, Ashley SE, Nash AG, et al. Timing of surgery in breast cancer. Lancet 1991; 337:1604.

26. Gnant MFX, Seifert M, Jakesz R, et al. Breast cancer and timing of surgery during menstrual cycle. A 5-year analysis of 385 premenopausal women. Int J Cancer 1992; 52:707-712.

27. Marques LA, Franco EL. Association between timing of surgery during menstrual cycle and prognosis in premenopausal breast cancer. Int J Cancer 1993; 53:707-708.

28. Ville Y, Briere M, Lasry S, et al. Timing of surgery in breast cancer. Lancet 1991; 337:1604-1605.

29. McGuire WL. The optimal timing of mastectomy: low tide or high tide? Ann Intern Med 1991; 115:401-403.

30. McGuire WL, Hilsenbeck S, Clark GM. Optimal mastectomy timing. J Natl Cancer Inst 1992; 48:346-348.

CHAPTER 11

CONCLUDING REMARKS

The concept of breast cancer as a disease which becomes systemic at a very early stage in its natural history has been validated by the prospective randomized trials of breast conservation therapy. Many women who might otherwise have been subjected to radical surgery have been treated conservatively without prejudice in terms of survival or disease-specific mortality. Adjuvant chemotherapy and endocrine manipulation have made modest inroads into the problems of breast cancer metastasis and mortality, but much remains to be done in this area.

Recent experience with preoperative adjuvant chemotherapy in locoregionally advanced and inflammatory breast cancer has quite possibly laid the foundation for another epochal advance in the management of breast cancer in the future. A number of studies have shown that aggressive preoperative chemotherapy results in partial and complete tumor responses in 70% to 90% of patients with locally advanced, nonmetastatic breast carcinoma. Moreover, early analyses strongly suggest that disease-free and overall survival of such patients may be greatly improved by primary chemotherapy.[1-5]

Preoperative adjuvant chemotherapy has also been used to downstage tumors of over 3 cm prior to undertaking breast-conserving surgery and radiotherapy.[6]

Others have postulated that it might eventually be possible to employ chemotherapy as the primary treatment modality, with radiotherapy for definitive control of the primary cancer and surgery held in reserve for local failure.[7-10] Developments such as the advent of recombinant colony-stimulating factors and autologous bone marrow transplantation have made high-dose chemotherapy trials feasible, and hold forth the hope that a major improvement in breast cancer cure rates may be within reach in the medium-term future. The effects that such an advance would have on current notions about locoregional breast cancer treatment are difficult to predict, but it is not inconceivable that surgery and/or radiotherapy could be relegated to a salvage or palliative role only.

Breast cancer prevention holds great promise for the future. Tamoxifen is only the first of perhaps many agents to be tested for chemopreventive activity in women at risk for breast cancer. Research in breast cancer genetics and molecular biology may well prove fruitful in this area as well.

The oncology community can take some momentary, modest satisfaction in the progress in understanding breast cancer biology over the past 20 years. While advances in locoregional and adjuvant systemic treatment have not translated into a major reduction in breast cancer mortality, they were often made in the face of fierce opposition from those who held to Halsted's concept of the behavior of breast cancer. The establishment of breast-conserving therapy as equal to radical surgery has been no mean feat, but the dividends have made the effort worthwhile. The morbidity and psychic burdens of treatment have been mitigated by breast conservation in a substantial proportion of patients afflicted with this disease.

REFERENCES

1. Sorace RA, Bagley CS, Lichter AS, et al. The management of nonmetastatic locally advanced breast cancer using primary induction chemotherapy with hormonal synchronization followed by radiation therapy with or without debulking surgery. World J Surg 1985; 9:775-785.

2. Rouëssé J, Friedman S, Sarrazin D, et al. Primary chemotherapy in the treatment of inflammatory carcinoma: a study of 230 cases from the Institut Gustave-Roussy. J Clin Oncol 1986; 4:1765-1771.

3. Hu E, Stockdale FE, Turner B, et al. Combined modality therapy of locally advanced breast cancer. Anticancer Res 1987; 7:733-736.

4. Swain SM, Sorace RA, Bagley CS, et al. Neoadjuvant chemotherapy in the combined modality approach of locally advanced nonmetastatic breast cancer. Cancer Res 1987; 47:3889-3894.

5. Schwartz GF, Cantor RI, Biermann WA. Neoadjuvant chemotherapy before definitive treatment for Stage III carcinoma of the breast. Arch Surg 1987; 122:1430-1434.

6. Bonadonna G, Veronesi U, Brambilla C, et al. Primary chemotherapy to avoid mastectomy in tumors with diameters of three centimeters or more. J Natl Cancer Inst 1990; 82:1539-1545.

7. Weil M, Borel Ch, Auclerc G, Baillet F, Khayat D. Nonsurgical approach in Stage I and Stage II breast cancer. Cancer Invest 1992; 10:581-586.

8. Bonadonna G. Conceptual and practical advances in the management of breast cancer. The Karnofsky Memorial Lecture. J Clin Oncol 1989; 7:1380-1397.

9. Ragaz J. Emerging modalities for adjuvant therapy of breast cancer: neoadjuvant chemotherapy. J Natl Cancer Inst Monogr 1986; 1:145-153.

10. Jacquillat C, Weil M, Baillet F, et al. Results of neoadjuvant chemotherapy and radiation therapy in the breast-conserving treatment of 250 patients with all stages of infiltrative breast cancer. Cancer 1990;66:119-129.

INDEX

DATE DUE

DEMCO 128-5046

(BC# 49571)

DEMCO